Orthopedic and Sports Medicine Case Studies for Nurse Practitioners

Karen M. Myrick, DNP, APRN, FNP-BC, ANP-BC, is a professor at Quinnipiac University with a joint appointment in the School of Nursing and the Frank Netter School of Medicine. She practices clinically as a nurse practitioner in Orthopedics and Sports Medicine in Glastonbury and Farmington, Connecticut, and her research focuses on athletes and sports medicine. The recipient of multiple grants, Dr. Myrick developed a newly designed physical examination technique for determining hip labral tears, The Hip Internal Rotation with Distraction (THIRD) test. In addition to publishing regularly in peer-reviewed journals, Dr. Myrick has written an academic book chapter on preventing childhood obesity. She is the senior editor of the *Journal of Clinical Case Reports*, and she recently received an award for Outstanding Poster at a national nurse practitioner conference for her work on "Recruiting and Retaining the Best and the Brightest Nurse Practitioner Faculty." (She has received several awards for Outstanding Poster at many other national conferences.) Dr. Myrick is the winner of the 2016 National Organizations of Nurse Practitioner Faculties (NONPF) Outstanding Researcher Award.

Orthopedic and Sports Medicine Case Studies for Nurse Practitioners

Karen M. Myrick, DNP, APRN, FNP-BC, ANP-BC

EDITOR

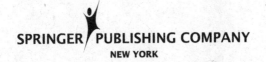

SPRINGER PUBLISHING COMPANY

NEW YORK

Springer Publishing Company, LLC
11 West 42nd Street
New York, NY 10036
www.springerpub.com

Acquisitions Editor: Margaret Zuccarini
Composition: diacriTech

ISBN: 978-0-8261-2253-7
e-book ISBN: 978-0-8261-2254-4
Instructor's Manual: 978-0-8261-2257-5

Instructor's Materials: Qualified instructors may request supplements by e-mailing textbook@springerpub.com

16 17 18 / 5 4 3 2 1

The author and the publisher of this Work have made every effort to use sources believed to be reliable to provide information that is accurate and compatible with the standards generally accepted at the time of publication. Because medical science is continually advancing, our knowledge base continues to expand. Therefore, as new information becomes available, changes in procedures become necessary. We recommend that the reader always consult current research and specific institutional policies before performing any clinical procedure. The author and publisher shall not be liable for any special, consequential, or exemplary damages resulting, in whole or in part, from the readers' use of, or reliance on, the information contained in this book. The publisher has no responsibility for the persistence or accuracy of URLs for external or third-party Internet websites referred to in this publication and does not guarantee that any content on such websites is, or will remain, accurate or appropriate.

Library of Congress Cataloging-in-Publication Data
Names: Myrick, Karen M., editor.
Title: Orthopedic and sports medicine case studies for nurse practitioners /
    Karen M. Myrick, editor.
Description: New York, NY : Springer Publishing Company, LLC, [2017] |
    Includes bibliographical references and index.
Identifiers: LCCN 2016020117| ISBN 9780826122537 | ISBN 9780826122575
    (instructors manual) | ISBN 9780826122544 (e-book)
Subjects: | MESH: Orthopedic Procedures | Sports Medicine—methods | Nurse
    Practitioners | Case Reports | Nurses' Instruction
Classification: LCC RD97 | NLM WE 168 | DDC 617.1/027—dc23 LC record available at
https://lccn.loc.gov/2016020117

Printed in the United States of America by McNaughton & Gunn.

This book is dedicated to my husband, Scott, and daughter, Kayden.
They keep me inspired and motivated.

Contents

SECTION III: SPINE CASES

Contributors

Jason N. DaCruz, MPAS, PA-C
Physician Assistant
Orthopedic Associates of Hartford
Hartford, Connecticut

Susan D'Agostino, DNP, APRN, FNP-BC
Assistant Professor of Nursing
Quinnipiac University
Hamden, Connecticut

Kevin Fitzsimmons, MHS, PA-C
Physician Assistant
Elite Sports Medicine
Connecticut Children's Medical Center
West Hartford, Connecticut

Kaitlin M. Ford, BS
Medical Student
Frank H. Netter School of Medicine
Quinnipiac University
Hamden, Connecticut

Phoebe M. Heffron, MSN, PPCNP-BC
Harvard, Massachusetts

Kimberly A. Joerg, DNP, APRN, PPCNP-BC
Assistant Professor of Nursing
University of St. Joseph
West Hartford, Connecticut

Teja Karukonda, MD
Resident
Department of Orthopedic Surgery
University of Connecticut
Farmington, Connecticut

Christine Kelly, MS, ATC
Athletic Training Resident
Elite Sports Medicine
Connecticut Children's Medical Center
West Hartford, Connecticut

Susan H. Lynch, DNP, APRN
Assistant Professor of Nursing
Quinnipiac University
Hamden, Connecticut

Karen M. Myrick, DNP, APRN, FNP-BC, ANP-BC
Assistant Professor of Nursing
Quinnipiac University
Hamden, Connecticut

Scott A. Myrick, MBA, AT, CSCS
Athletic Trainer and Certified Strength and Conditioning Specialist
Myrick Wealth Planning
Myrick Benefits Solutions
West Hartford, Connecticut

Karen M. Pawelek, DNP, APRN
Part-Time Faculty
Department of Nursing
University of South Dakota
Vermillion, South Dakota
Quinnipiac University
Hamden, Connecticut

Craig M. Rodner, MD
Associate Professor
Department of Orthopedic Surgery
University of Connecticut
Farmington, Connecticut

Vinayak M. Sathe, MD, MS, FRCS
Assistant Professor
Department of Orthopedic Surgery
University of Connecticut
Farmington, Connecticut

Hardeep Singh, MD
Resident
Department of Orthopedic Surgery
University of Connecticut
Farmington, Connecticut

Daniel Witmer, MD
Resident
Department of Orthopedic Surgery
University of Connecticut
Farmington, Connecticut

Foreword

The current book by Dr. Karen M. Myrick and associated authors titled *Orthopedic and Sports Medicine Case Studies for Nurse Practitioners* is timely, comprehensive and, perhaps most important, practical. As a practicing orthopedic sports medicine physician, I can unequivocally state that we rely heavily on well-trained nurse practitioners to provide comprehensive evaluation and care for our patients.

Whether it be in the office setting, emergency department, training room, or operating room setting, a knowledgeable and competent nurse practitioner is an invaluable member of the sports medicine team. This work greatly facilitates a practical learning experience and expands the fund of knowledge in a didactic format, but also in a case-based manner, which provides the reader with real-life scenarios for improved understanding and comprehension.

This work covers many common topics presenting to the office, training room, or emergency department involving the shoulder, elbow, wrist, hip, knee, and spine. There are several chapters addressing many acute injuries such as acute shoulder and elbow dislocation, patellar dislocation, and acute anterior cruciate ligament tears. There are also excellent chapters dedicated to chronic overuse problems such as patellar tendinopathy, lateral epicondylitis, and rotator cuff tendinitis, just to name several. The knowledge gained from expertise in these areas markedly improves patient care for athletes and active patients. Command of this information makes the nurse practitioner an outstanding clinician in an area where all too frequently there is a lack of even rudimentary skill in evaluating the orthopedic sports medicine patient.

In summary, the case-based approach has been well-recognized as one of the most beneficial methods of teaching. For the past several years, the American Academy of Orthopedic Surgery and the American Orthopedic Society of Sports Medicine have embraced this approach in teaching orthopedists, residents, and fellows at their annual meetings. Symposia and instructional courses utilizing this form of teaching "sell out" and are the most popular courses offered. Dr. Myrick and her colleagues have put together a textbook utilizing this approach to provide the most current state-of-the-art knowledge on myriad orthopedic sports medicine topics.

I am confident it will be a sought-after and extremely popular textbook, and will lead to other editions. This will be a most valuable resource for the nurse practitioner at any level.

Robert A. Arciero, MD
Professor, Orthopedics
President of the American Orthopedic Society for Sports Medicine, 2014–2015
Director, University of Connecticut Orthopedic Sports Medicine Fellowship
Team Physician, University of Connecticut
Storrs and Farmington, Connecticut

Preface

We hope you find this work an educational resource, and enjoy *Orthopedic and Sports Medicine Case Studies for Nurse Practitioners*. This text offers a significant contribution to the existing market, filling a gap that has been identified by students, professors, and practitioners alike. There is a paucity of case studies in the field of orthopedics and sports medicine. This work can assist in the preparation of nurse practitioners for treating patients with orthopedic and sports medicine injuries and conditions. Furthermore, there is a lack of cases in the specialty specifically written *by* nurse practitioners who are also professors *for* nurse practitioners and professors.

The main theme of the book is to provide challenging case studies in the specialty of orthopedics and sports medicine. These cases follow a template that is designed to provide students with a meaningful learning experience as they critically think about answers to the case questions. The case studies also allow the instructor to work the cases both inductively and deductively. Many facts about specific conditions and injuries are included.

The objective of the book is to provide orthopedic and sports medicine case studies that are clinically relevant for nurse practitioners. Following a pattern of faculty-identified affinity for case studies, the book provides a useful resource for teaching in this specialty area.

The distinguishing elements include the less common area of orthopedics and sports medicine specific cases. Information for both acute care and primary care are included, identifying cases that are likely to be encountered in each of the distinguished areas in clinical practice.

The book is intended for nurse practitioner students and nurse practitioner faculty. The book can be used at the master's or doctoral level of preparation, and is intended to teach the specialty of orthopedics and sports medicine. The programs include all nurse practitioner preparation programs, including courses in health assessment, primary and acute care, and common and/or complex problems. Clinical seminar courses could also choose to adopt the book to enhance clinical experiences. **Qualified instructors can obtain an Instructor's Manual to accompany this text by e-mailing Springer Publishing Company at textbook@springerpub.com.**

Karen M. Myrick

Acknowledgments

Thank you, Alyssa Bozzuto, RT(R), at Orthopedic Associates, for your attention to detail, and willingness to assist in this important work.

SECTION I

Upper Extremity Cases

CHAPTER 1

Shoulder

Case Study 1.1: Traumatic Shoulder Dislocation

Scott A. Myrick and Karen M. Myrick

SETTING: URGENT CARE

Definition and Incidence

The estimated incidence of shoulder dislocations in the United States is approximately 24 per 100,000 person-years (Zacchilli & Owens, 2010). Person-years is the product of the number of years times the number of members of a population who have been affected by a certain condition. Furthermore, young age and male sex are risk factors for shoulder dislocation (Zacchilli & Owens, 2010). Athletes who participate in contact and collision sports are at a higher risk.

Patient

A 35-year-old male presents with a chief complaint of left shoulder pain and a feeling that his shoulder "went out." The patient was playing a pick-up game of lacrosse in a local men's league after work. He reached up high with his stick to catch a pass and was hit from the front and side by another player and landed face down on the turf. After landing on the ground, another player fell on his outstretched arm and he immediately had a feeling of weakness and intense pain in his shoulder. The pain is a 9 out of 10, 10 being most painful, and there is no associated numbness or tingling. Pain is exacerbated when he is not supporting the arm at the elbow, and seems to radiate down to his wrist.

Social History

The patient is an active former collegiate lacrosse player. He drives a forklift at a local manufacturing plant full time. His work includes moving heavy boxes and stacking them onto pallets. He does not currently smoke, and drinks a couple nights a week. He is single, and does not have any children.

> **CLINICAL PEARL**
>
> The most prudent course of treatment for a first time traumatic dislocation is surgical repair to stabilize the joint and repair any damage to assure best patient outcomes. When suspecting a shoulder dislocation, three radiographic views should be obtained, an anterior–posterior view, axillary view, and transscapular lateral view (also referred to as a "Y" view) (see Figure 1.1). These allow for the visualization of a Hill-Sachs lesion and may suggest the presence of a Bankart lesion (tear of the anterior labrum) (see Figure 1.2). Bankart lesions are the most common type of complication with anterior shoulder dislocations (Kim, Cho, Son, & Moon, 2014).

Physical Assessment

He stands 6'2", 185 lb, with an athletic build. He is in great distress due to the shoulder pain. He is neurologically intact. Capillary refill as measured is brisk. On palpation, there is a marked step off, distal to the acromion.

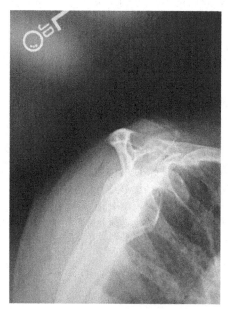

FIGURE 1.1 Y-scapular radiographic view of shoulder dislocation.

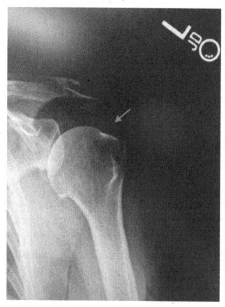

FIGURE 1.2 Radiograph of the shoulder demonstrating a Hill-Sach's deformity.

Additional palpation reveals diffuse pain and spasm in the musculature surrounding the shoulder joint. When asked to perform active range of motion (ROM), the patient attempts forward flexion but is unable to move the arm due to pain. Passively he allows his arm to reach approximately 50 degrees of forward flexion. In light of the significant limitations in his ROM and high level of pain, strength testing is not performed, nor are any special tests.

Diagnostic Evaluations

A radiograph was obtained to look for the presence of any fracture, and to evaluate the position of the humeral head. There is no visible evidence of any fracture but a Hill-Sachs lesion is clearly shown. The views also demonstrate an anterior dislocation, and a positive "empty glenoid" sign, as demonstrated in Figure 1.3.

Diagnosis

Left anterior shoulder dislocation with Hill-Sachs lesion.

Interventions

Dislocations are frightening to the patient, and reassurance is the first course of treatment. Explaining in plain terms that you will be attempting to reduce the shoulder quickly, it is important for the patient to understand and cooperate as best he can. After explaining this route to him, he elects, signs consent, and is placed prone without his shirt on a treatment table. A nerve

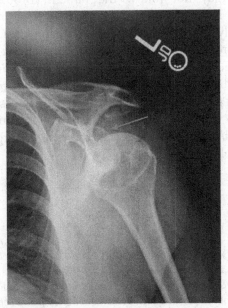

FIGURE 1.3 Radiograph demonstrating the "empty glenoid" sign with anterior shoulder dislocation.

block is performed with 6 mL of Marcaine and 2 mL of lidocaine injected with a posterior approach distal to the acromion. This is met with some pain relief by the patient.

Next, the patient assumes a supine position with a therapy belt under his left axilla where a counter force is applied toward the patient's left ear. Then, a traction force is applied to the patient's left arm by gripping the distal wrist in a direction directly opposite that of the therapy belt. While an initial small force is applied, the shoulder should slip back into place with the cooperation of a relaxed patient.

Once the reduction is complete, the patient is placed in a sling with pillow attachment, which would allow him a comfortable resting position. He is instructed on a regimen of nonsteroidal anti-inflammatory drugs (NSAIDs) and icing four to six times daily. Lastly, follow-up with an orthopedist is advised within the next 1 to 3 days. Postreduction radiographs are obtained.

Patient Education

It is important to educate the patient that first-time anterior shoulder dislocations are best treated with surgical stabilization. Given this, it's important the patient understands how preferable the outcomes with surgical treatment are versus nonsurgical treatment.

Follow-Up Evaluation

As this injury will most likely require surgical consultation, the nurse practitioner may not follow the patient through his entire continuum of care. If the nurse practitioner is in a setting where nurses work collaboratively with an orthopedic surgeon, the nurse may refer the patient if there is no initial progress being made or simply collaborate on the most effective course of treatment. For the primary care nurse practitioner, it is likely the patient would return after rehabilitation has been completed in order to gauge the athlete's readiness to return to his sport. This may be done in conjunction and collaboration with the physical therapist and/or athletic trainer. In the case of surgery, the surgeon may oversee the follow-up.

REFERENCES

Kim, Y., Cho, S., Son, W., & Moon, S. (2014). Arthroscopic repair of small and medium-sized Bony Bankart lesions. *American Journal of Sports Medicine, 42*(1), 86–94.

Zacchilli, M. A., & Owens, B. D. (2010). Epidemiology of shoulder dislocations presenting to emergency departments in the United States. *Journal of Bone & Joint Surgery, 92*(3), 542–549. doi:10.2106/JBJS.I.00450

Case Study 1.2: Acute Acromioclavicular Separation

Karen M. Myrick

SETTING: URGENT CARE

Definition and Incidence

Acromioclavicular (AC) separations are commonly known as "shoulder separations." As a common injury, AC separation affects patients at all age groups across the life span (Wright, MacLeod, & Talwalker, 2011).

Patient

Patient presents with the chief complaint of left shoulder pain. There was an acute onset of pain when the patient slipped on ice, landing directly onto the left shoulder and left side this morning. Pain is rated as 6 out of 10, aching in quality, relieved slightly with ibuprofen 800 mg and keeping his arm supported at the elbow. Pain is not associated with any numbness or tingling or other symptoms.

Social History

This 37-year-old male is an accountant and father of three young children ages 6, 7, and 9. He is active with running and martial arts training.

> **CLINICAL PEARL**
>
> Depending on the degree of the AC separation, surgical intervention might be indicated (Felder & Mair, 2015). AC separations are graded I to VI, with I being the least degree of damage and displacement, and VI being complete disruption of the acromioclavicular and coracoclavicular ligaments (see Table 1.1).

Physical Assessment

The patient is a 37-year-old male who is in no acute distress, but demonstrates hesitancy and some discomfort throughout the physical examination. He is 5'10" and weighs 186 lb. He has an obvious step off at the AC joint to inspection, and tenderness over the AC joint with palpation. He has an intact shoulder shrug with examination, clavicle rising on both the left and the right sides. Shoulder range of motion is full, but uncomfortable throughout motion. There are no focal neurological deficits in the left upper extremity.

Diagnostic Evaluations

A radiograph was obtained, and demonstrates widening of the AC joint consistent with a type II AC separation (see Figure 1.4).

CLINICAL PEARL

If the shoulder shrug is intact with equal rising on both sides, this indicates that the deltoid and trapezius muscles are intact.

TABLE 1.1 Degrees of Acromioclavicular Separation

I. Acromioclavicular ligament sprain
II. Acromioclavicular ligament disrupted
III. Acromioclavicular and coracoclavicular ligaments disrupted
IV. Acromioclavicular and coracoclavicular ligaments disrupted and distal (lateral) clavicle displaced posteriorly
V. Acromioclavicular and coracoclavicular ligaments disrupted, attachments of deltoid and trapezious murcleson clavicle disrupted, clavicle displaces superiorly
VI. Acromioclavicular and coracoclavicular ligaments disrupted, clavicle displaces inferiorly

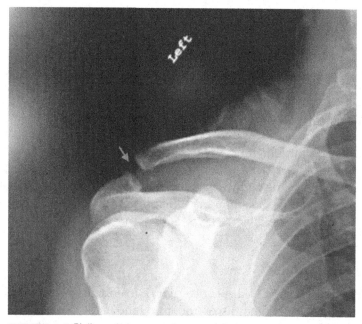

FIGURE 1.4 Radiograph demonstrating second-degree acromioclavicular separation.

Diagnosis

Type II AC separation.

Interventions

The patient was placed into a sling for comfort, and a 2-week follow-up visit was recommended. Modalities for decreasing inflammation such as a NSAIDs, ice 20 minutes three times a day, and rest were recommended.

Patient Education

The elbow is one of the joints in the body that may become stiff very quickly. Although recommending a sling and using it for comfort is good practice, it is important to recommend that the patient also take the arm out of the sling five to seven times a day and perform full elbow range of motion.

Follow-Up Evaluation

At the 2-week follow-up visit, the patient was relating the decreased use of the sling on most occasions, as his discomfort was significantly less at this point. The step off was decreased on evaluation, and shoulder range of motion was full, but now without discomfort except for the extremes of motion. Six-week course of physical therapy was recommended, and follow-up on an as-needed basis after that.

REFERENCES

Felder, J. J., & Mair, S. D. (2015). Acromioclavicular joint injuries. *Current Orthopaedic Practice, 26*(2), 113–118.

Wright, A., MacLeod, I., & Talwalker, S. (2011). Disorders of the acromioclavicular joint and distal clavicle. *Orthopaedics & Trauma, 25*(1), 30–36. doi:10.1016/.jmporth.2010.10.011

Case Study 1.3: Acute Rupture of the Biceps Tendon

Scott A. Myrick

SETTING: URGENT CARE

Definition and Incidence

The distal biceps tendon is the primary supinator of the elbow, and a strong flexor of the elbow (Virk, DiVenere, & Mazzocca, 2014). Injuries to this area are typically traumatic in nature whereas overuse or chronic injuries of the biceps tendon usually occur proximally at the shoulder joint.

Patient

The patient is a 46-year-old male dump truck operator who presents with the chief complaint of right shoulder pain and deformity. He describes a history where earlier in the day he was driving on an icy road. He lost control of the vehicle and as he tried to right the truck, which was sliding into a ditch, the force of the steering wheel caused his arm to move in a quick and awkward manner. He describes feeling a pop and immediate pain in the "crease" of his elbow. The discomfort has subsided slightly from his initial pain, which was a 9 out of 10 to a level of 5 out of 10, 10 being most painful. The patient complains of no other ailments, neck or shoulder pain, and denies any numbness or tingling in this right upper extremity. According to the patient, he has had no prior injuries to his extremities nor has he been out of work for any reason other than illness.

Social History

This 46-year-old male works for a transportation company. Duties of his job involve not only driving trucks but also assisting with unloading cargo. He is employed full time, working long days.

He is an overweight male with a history of smoking. The patient describes himself as a social drinker who has an affinity for cars. He does not exercise and is primarily sedentary both in his job and outside. Given the nature of his employment, it's evident this particular injury will impact his ability to perform his job and he will need to be placed on light duty or possibly on workman's compensation.

CLINICAL PEARL

Distal biceps tendon tears are more common in men and in their fourth decade of life (Kelly, Perkinson, Ablove, & Tueting, 2015).

Physical Assessment

Presentation of the patient shows no acute distress. He is 5'8" and weighs 230 lb. When greeting the patient, he does shake hands willingly, although tentatively. Upon examination of the affected elbow, inspection demonstrates the "Popeye" deformity that is common with this injury (Figure 1.5). With palpation, there is mild swelling apparent along with a palpable "step off" just proximal to the insertion of the distal biceps tendon on the proximal radius.

Range of motion is full extension with the patient describing a feeling of stiffness at full extension, and 120 degrees of flexion passively, inhibited by pain. Strength testing reveals pain with both flexion and extension, and 3 out of 5 strength with flexion and 2 out of 5 strength with supination. With ligamentous testing of the elbow, both varus and valgus stress testing is normal with minimal gap and a tight end feel, at both 0 and 30 degrees of flexion. Neurologically, the patient has normal sensation throughout the length of his affected arm.

Diagnostic Evaluations

A radiograph was not obtained, due to the lack of yield on information that would be likely in this patient. Although considered, an MRI was not obtained, as the history and physical examination of the patient is highly specific for the diagnosis of torn distal biceps tendon.

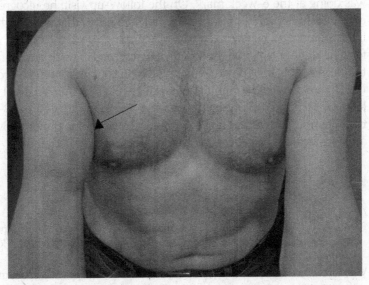

FIGURE 1.5 The "popeye" deformity that is commonly demonstrated with a biceps tendon rupture.

Diagnosis

Distal biceps tendon tear.

Interventions

The patient was educated on the RICE treatment (rest, ice, compression, and elevation). Specifically, the patient was told to rest his arm from aggravating movements, ice four to six times daily for 20 minutes each time, lightly wrapping his elbow with a compression bandage to help with swelling, and to elevate the arm as much as possible. He was also instructed on a regimen of NSAIDs to be taken daily with food; Naprosyn 500 mg twice a day with food was recommended

Lastly, a routine of physical therapy was prescribed two to three times a week for 6 weeks, with a focus on strengthening the musculature both proximal and distal to the elbow joint as well as postural muscles surrounding the shoulder joint.

Patient Education

It is very important to educate the patient about the possible treatment options for treatment of bicep tendon tears, which include operative and nonoperative management. This is important in helping the patient make the decision about electing for either surgical or nonsurgical intervention and in identifying the likelihood that the Popeye deformity will be permanent without surgery, as well as result in some loss in supination strength.

Follow-Up Evaluation

This patient opted to try a nonoperative course of treatment, and to see how he was doing at the 6-week mark. On the follow-up visit, he recognized that the deformity in his right upper arm was not something that was worthy of surgical intervention, and he wanted a trial of returning to work to see if he could perform his duties with enough strength. He returned to work, and was encouraged to return for his final physical therapy visit to obtain a home exercise program (HEP) that he would continue to maximize his strength, in light of his torn distal biceps tendon. Follow-up was arranged for 3 months. At the 3-month visit, the patient reported that he could, in fact, perform his duties and his daily life activities without pain, and he was released from care at that time.

REFERENCES

Kelly, M., Perkinson, S., Ablove, R., & Tueting, J. (2015). Distal biceps tendon ruptures. *American Journal of Sports Medicine* [serial online], 43(8), 2012–2017. Retrieved from *SPORTDiscus with full text*, Ipswich, MA.

Virk, M. S., DiVenere, J., & Mazzocca, A. D. (2014). Distal biceps tendon injuries: Treatment of partial and complete tears. *Operative Techniques in Sports Medicine*, 22(2), 156–163.

Case Study 1.4: Chronic Rotator Cuff Tendinitis

Karen M. Myrick

SETTING: PRIMARY CARE

Definition and Incidence

Rotator cuff tendinitis is a common condition, and the pathophysiology that is causative is not well understood (Kolk, Yang, Tamminga, & van der Hoeven, 2013). Shoulder injuries are one of the most commonly seen in primary care and orthopedic clinics (Kim, Kang, Kim, & Oh, 2014).

Patient

Patient presents with the chief complaint of right shoulder pain for the past several months. The pain is worse when he does overhead work, and wakes him up four out of seven nights a week when he rolls onto that side. He describes the discomfort as aching in quality, and sharp with certain sudden movements, such as reaching a bag out of the car, or a suitcase from an overhead bin. Discomfort is well located in the right shoulder, and does not radiate down the arm. Pain is rated as a 2 out of 10, and when the sharp discomfort occurs, it is a 7 to 8 out of 10. He tried ibuprofen, 800 mg three times a day for the last week, but really did not find this to make a difference in the discomfort. He has had to modify his workout routine with resistance training, and has had to stop swimming. He has not tried applying ice or heat.

Social History

This 47-year-old male is a baseball coach and teacher at the local university. He is in the off-season for his sport, but keeps active to maintain his fitness, weight, and to control his cholesterol and hypertension. He travels occasionally on business to recruit athletes for his team.

CLINICAL PEARL

Asking a patient if the pain awakens him or her at night is a good way to identify the impact on a patient's activities of daily living, and a guide to help evaluate improvement in his or her condition.

Physical Assessment

The patient is a 47-year-old male who is in no acute distress, but demonstrates hesitancy and some discomfort throughout the physical examination. He is 6'4" and weighs 219 lb. On inspection, there is no obvious deformity and shoulders appear to be equal in size and muscle bulk. There are no open cuts or abrasions, no rashes or lesions. With palpation, there is some mild tenderness with palpation of the biceps tendon in the bicipital groove but no bony tenderness is appreciated. Neck range of motion is full, and there is no provocation of his symptoms with motion of the neck. A Spurling maneuver is negative. Shoulder range of motion in forward elevation is 0 to 180 degrees actively, with pain from 110 to 180. Internal rotation is just to the waist on his right shoulder, which is five vertebral bodies less than the contralateral left, unaffected side. Passive range of motion reveals a positive impingement sign, with pain from 130 to 170 degrees. There is a negative drop arm test, but any strength testing of the supraspinatus causes him discomfort. Strength testing is 4 out of 5 with the supraspinatus test, and seemingly inhibited by discomfort. He has a negative sulcus test, and negative lift-off sign. There are no focal neurological deficits in the right upper extremity.

> ### CLINICAL PEARL
>
> Always be certain to rule out the neck as a cause of shoulder pain. Cervical radiculopathy can complicate the patient presentation.

Diagnostic Evaluations

A radiograph was not obtained, due to the lack of yield on information that would be likely in this patient. If symptoms were still present at the 6-week follow-up after treatment, radiographs should be obtained.

Diagnosis

Rotator cuff tendinitis.

Interventions

The patient was encouraged to limit overhead activities until follow-up, and return in 6 weeks for evaluation. Physical therapy was ordered at a frequency of two to three times a week for the next 6 weeks. He was continued on his regimen of 800 mg of ibuprofen with food, three times a day.

Patient Education

Strengthening the rotator cuff is one of the key suggestions by clinicians in rotator cuff tendinitis intervention programs (Kim et al., 2014). It is also important to maintain a good posture, with shoulders retracted and head well centered over the cervical spine.

Follow-Up Evaluation

At the follow-up visit, the patient was not feeling much improvement. He reported waking two out of seven nights a week with discomfort, and continued inability to swim and continued necessary modifications in his weight-lifting routine. At this point, a discussion is held with the patient about treatment options. He is offered an injection with cortisone and Marcaine, with the information that most clinicians agree to the limit of no more than three injections in a joint in a lifetime. Because his baseball season is coming up, and he expects to be pain free and be able to throw with his athletes, he chooses to have the injection. He tolerates this very well, and he returns in 6 months for evaluation. At this time, he is no longer experiencing any discomfort, except when he "overdoes it," and he has continued the exercises taught in physical therapy to strengthen the rotator cuff and surrounding musculature.

CLINICAL PEARL

Patients frequently need to be reminded to continue their exercises once their formal physical therapy sessions have been completed. A HEP is typically provided to the patient.

REFERENCES

Kim, S., Kang, M., Kim, E., & Oh, J. (2014). Kinesio taping improves shoulder internal rotation and the external/internal rotator strength ratio in patients with rotator cuff tendinitis. *Isokinetics & Exercise Science, 22*(3), 259–263.

Kolk, A., Yang, K. G., Tamminga, R., & van der Hoeven, H. (2013). Radial extracorporeal shock-wave therapy in patients with chronic rotator cuff tendinitis: A prospective randomised double-blind placebo-controlled multicentre trial. *Bone & Joint Journal, 95-B*(11), 1521–1526. doi:10.1302/0301-620X.95B11.31879

Case Study 1.5: Chronic Osteoarthritis

Karen M. Pawelek

SETTING: PRIMARY CARE

Definition and Incidence

Osteoarthritis (OA) is defined as a "joint failure" due to pathologic changes in a joint over time (Kasper, Fauci, Longo, Jameson, & Lascalzo, 2015). In chronic OA of the shoulder, the glenoid labrum and humeral head articular cartilage undergoes pathologic changes (Kasper et al., 2015). OA of the shoulder is relatively uncommon when compared to weight-bearing joints such as the knee, hip, and fingers. It tends to be more common in women older than the age of 60 and is most often the result of trauma (Nakagawa, Hyakuna, Otani, Hashitani, & Nakamura, 1999). Oftentimes, the trauma occurs several years preceding the onset of symptoms.

The types of trauma that are most often associated with chronic shoulder OA include a previous dislocation, fracture of the humeral head or neck, or a rotator cuff tear (Nakagawa et al., 1999). Another cause of OA may result from the detachment of the superior glenoid labrum from the anterior to posterior aspect (SLAP) (Patzer, Lichtenberg, Kircher, Magosch, & Habermeyer, 2010).

Patient

Patient presents with pain in the right shoulder. Initially she noticed the pain in her right shoulder approximately 1 month ago and it has progressively been getting worse. The pain feels like a "deep" pressure in her shoulder and is mainly present with movement or pressure of the area. She describes the pain as a 6 out of 10 when present. Pain is not worse at night or first thing in the morning. She has never had this pain before, but in the past she did have a shoulder dislocation once in the same shoulder. Occasionally the pain radiated to her right neck area, but not beyond. She has tried 650 mg Tylenol once daily at bedtime for the past week, but has noticed no difference. She has also tried ice alternating with heat a few times with some improvement. Generally, she avoided moving the arm in order to limit the pain for the past few days.

Social History

She played tennis for many years, but stopped a few years ago. She prefers walking 20 minutes per day most days, drinks one to two glasses of wine daily, is married, and lives with her husband.

Physical Assessment

The patient is a 75-year-old female who presents in no acute distress: shoulders symmetrical on inspection without obvious deformity. With palpation, she has tenderness and crepitus along right acromioclavicular (AC) joint. The patient demonstrates a positive right cross-over adduction test. She also has pain with AC resistance testing. She is neurovascularly intact distal to the shoulder in the right arm without any focal deficits.

Diagnostic Evaluations

Anterioposterior, lateral and axial views of the shoulder are obtained. These demonstrate mild joint space narrowing of the glenohumeral and of the AC joint. There is evidence of osteophyte formation at the glenoid (see Figure 1.6).

Diagnosis

Degenerative arthritis of the shoulder, including the glenohumeral and acromioclavicular joint.

Interventions

NSAIDs for pain control was recommended initially since the patient had no prior history of bleeding risks or kidney disease. Once the pain subsided, the patient performed pendulum exercises at least three times a day after a demonstration in the office was provided. The patient was instructed to take a warm shower for 10 to 15 minutes prior to performing the pendulum exercises. Physical therapy for individualized exercise plan was also recommended, as well as avoidance of activities that elicit pain (overhead and cross-body movement) until symptoms improved; then gradually, added usual back activities were also recommended.

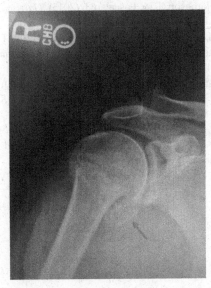

FIGURE 1.6 Radiograph of the right shoulder demonstrating osteoarthritis with osteophyte formation.

Patient Education

Importantly, educate your patient that a trial of scheduled acetaminophen may be used if there is no relief with NSAIDs (Zhang, Jones, & Doherty, 2004). If there is no relief after NSAIDs and/or acetaminophen, a glucocorticoid injection may provide relief.

Once the pain has resolved, rotator cuff strengthening exercises should be initiated.

Follow-Up Evaluation

The patient was encouraged to return in 3 months for a follow-up visit to assess symptoms and range of motion. At this point a repeat x-ray was obtained to assess for disease progression. Referral to surgery may be an option if the symptoms are not improved with conservative measures.

This patient gradually improved and became more functional in terms of her right upper extremity range of motion. She continued to use acetaminophen intermittently and continued with the exercises advised by the physical therapist.

The patient asked about alternative therapies such as chondroitin and glucosamine. She was advised this was not supported by the literature or the Food and Drug Administration (FDA), but if she chose to do a trial on these over-the-counter products, she should purchase them from a reputable company. She should also make it known to any health care provider that she was using these products.

REFERENCES

Kasper, D., Fauci, A., Longo, D., Jameson, J., & Lascalzo, J. (2015). *Harrison's principles of internal medicine* (19th ed.). New York, NY: McGraw-Hill.

Nakagawa, Y., Hyakuna, K., Otani, S., Hashitani, M., & Nakamura, T. (1999). Epidemiologic study of glenohumeral osteoarthritis with plain radiography. *Journal of Shoulder, Elbow Surgery, 9*(6), 580–584.

Patzer, T., Lichtenberg, S., Kircher, J., Magosch, P., & Habermeyer, P. (2010). Influence of SLAP lesions on chondral lesions of the glenohumeral joint. *Knee Surgery, Sports Traumatology, Arthroscopy, 18*(7), 982–987.

Zhang, W., Jones, A., & Doherty, M. (2004). Does paracetamol (acetaminophen) reduce the pain of osteoarthritis? A meta-analysis of randomised controlled trials. *Annual of Rheumatology Disease, 63*(8), 901–907.

Case Study 1.6: Chronic Calcific Tendinitis

Karen M. Myrick

SETTING: PRIMARY CARE

Definition and Incidence

As a common continuation of rotator cuff tendinitis, calcific tendinitis is a possible intraarticular condition. It is thought that rotator cuff tendinitis caused by degenerative changes is replaced by fibrocartilage, which then calcifies (Kolk, Yang, Tamminga, & van der Hoeven, 2013).

Patient

Patient presents with the chief complaint of left shoulder pain for the past year and a half. Pain is constantly present, and wakes her up seven nights a week when she rolls onto that side. She has seen two orthopedic providers, and has gone to two separate 6-week sessions of physical therapy in the last year. She received a cortisone injection into this left shoulder 8 weeks ago, which initially helped to decrease the pain, and lasted approximately 3 weeks. She is frustrated that she is not getting better, and describes the discomfort as aching in quality, and very sharp with certain sudden movements, such as doing her hair, and it has become impossible to hook her bra behind her back. Discomfort does not radiate down the arm. Pain is rated as a 4 out of 10, and when the sharp discomfort occurs, it is a 9 out of 10. She has been on a regimen of Naprosyn 500 mg twice a day for the past 6 to 8 months, and this initially helped with her pain for the first couple of months, but it is no longer effective.

> ### CLINICAL PEARL
>
> The pain associated with rotator cuff tendinitis is typically worse with activity, whereas the pain associated with calcific tendinitis is not characteristically activity dependent (Wolf, 1999).

Social History

This 51-year-old female is a legal secretary at a local law firm. She has two adult children in college.

Physical Assessment

The patient is a 51-year-old female in no acute distress, but has discomfort throughout the physical examination especially with range of motion. She is 5'5" and weighs 151 lb. On inspection, there is no obvious deformity and shoulders appear to be equal in size and bulk without any atrophy. There are no open cuts or abrasions, no rashes or lesions. With palpation, there is some mild tenderness throughout the shoulder, without specific tenderness at any key landmarks. Neck range of motion is full, and there is no aggravation of her symptoms throughout. A Spurling maneuver is performed and is negative. Shoulder range of motion in forward elevation is 0 to 150 degrees actively, with pain from 120 to 150. Internal rotation is not possible, and causes discomfort. A positive impingement sign is identified with passive motion and pain from 130 to 150 degrees. There is a negative drop arm test. Strength testing of the supraspinatus causes her significant discomfort. Strength testing is 3 out of 5 with the suprispinatous test, inhibited as soon as she feels discomfort. She has a negative sulcus test, and negative lift-off sign. There are no focal neurological deficits in the left upper extremity.

Diagnostic Evaluations

A radiograph was obtained, and demonstrated calcific tendinitis in the left shoulder (Figure 1.7).

Diagnosis

Calcific tendinitis, left shoulder

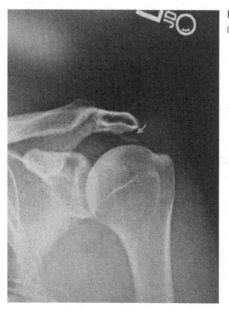

FIGURE 1.7 Radiograph of the left shoulder demonstrating calcific tendinitis.

Interventions

This patient has undergone the conservative treatment options for rotator cuff calcific tendinitis. At this point, it is prudent to refer to an orthopedic specialist for further evaluation and treatment.

CLINICAL PEARL

The treatment options vary and typically begin with the least invasive to more invasive for most orthopedic conditions, and take a stepwise approach. In this case, the initial options include what she has tried (anti-inflammatory medications, physical therapy, and activity modifications). The moderately invasive steroid injection has not helped her either and this is indication for surgical intervention with arthroscopic needling and aspiration of the calcific deposit (Wolf, 1999).

Patient Education

Strengthening the rotator cuff is one of the key suggestions by clinicians in rotator cuff tendinitis intervention programs (Yoo, 2010). With the calcific deposit, often physical therapy and strengthening is not sufficient to alleviate discomfort, and injections with corticosteroids or surgical intervention are recommended.

Follow-Up Evaluation

At the follow-up visit, the patient was not feeling much improvement. She reported awakening two out of seven nights with discomfort, and continued inability to be able to perform her activities of daily living without significant discomfort. At this point, she was referred to an orthopedic surgeon for possible surgical intervention, for arthroscopic evaluation and debridement of the calcific deposit, and possible subacromial decompression and distal clavicle excision.

REFERENCES

Kolk, A., Yang, K. G., Tamminga, R., & van der Hoeven, H. (2013). Radial extracorporeal shock-wave therapy in patients with chronic rotator cuff tendinitis: A prospective randomised double-blind placebo-controlled multicentre trial. *Bone & Joint Journal*, 95-B(11), 1521–1526. doi:10.1302/0301-620X.95B11.31879

Wolf, W. (1999). Calcific tendinitis of the shoulder: Diagnosis and simple, effective treatment. [Tendinite calcifiante des courts rotateurs de l'épaule. Diagnostic et traitement simple et efficace]. *Physician & Sportsmedicine, 27*(9), 27–33.

Yoo, J., Park, W., Koh, K., & Kim, S. (2010). Arthroscopic treatment of chronic calcific tendinitis with complete removal and rotator cuff tendon repair. *Knee Surgery, Sports Traumatology, Arthroscopy, 18*(12), 1694–1699. doi:10.1007/s00167-010-1067-7

CHAPTER **2**

Elbow

Case Study 2.1: Acute Elbow Dislocation

Christine Kelly

SETTING: EMERGENCY DEPARTMENT FOLLOWED UP AT SPORTS MEDICINE CLINIC

Definition and Incidence

The elbow is the second most commonly dislocated major joint in the general population and the fifth most commonly injured body part in young athletes (Adirim & Cheng, 2003; Dizdarevic et al., 2015). The National Electronic Injury Surveillance System database demonstrates the highest incidence of elbow dislocations occurring between the ages of 10 and 19, with sports participation being the most frequent cause of injury (Stoneback et al., 2012). The elbow is a hinge joint that relies heavily on the congruency of the distal humerus and proximal ulna for stability. There are three joint articulations that make up the elbow: humeroulnar, humeroradial, and radioulnar. These three joints allow for elbow flexion, extension, pronation, and supination. An elbow dislocation typically occurs from falling on an outstretched hand (FOOSH), with the forearm supinated, wrist extended, and the elbow flexed 20 degrees or less. This mechanism causes an axial load toward the elbow joint, increasing stress across the surrounding ligamentous structures, and ultimately leads to a potential dislocation event. Dislocations are classified in the direction of movement: anterior, posterior, medial, or lateral, with posterolateral being the most common direction for elbow dislocations. Elbow dislocations are also described as either simple (no fracture) or complex (evidence of fracture).

Patient

Patient is an 11-year-old, left-hand-dominant male.

Social History

Patient is an 11-year-old, left-hand-dominant male, who has no pertinent past medical or surgical history and no previous injuries to his elbow. He is active and participates in football.

Physical Assessment

He presents to the emergency department (ED) with a chief complaint of right elbow pain. The patient described an event while playing running back in a football game. He was running with the ball in his left hand, was tackled and fell to the ground onto an outstretched right upper extremity. He experienced immediate pain with obvious deformity noted at the right elbow. Upon arrival to the ED, the patient reported moderate pain with guarding of his right elbow at approximately 90 degrees of flexion. On physical exam, obvious deformity of the humeroulnar joint was seen and felt, the presence of a distal radial pulse was felt, skin appeared pink and warm, and the patient had normal sensory distribution of the radial, median, and ulnar nerves, with intact motor function along the distribution of his anterior interosseous, posterior interosseous, and ulnar nerves. He demonstrated minimal range of motion (ROM) at the right wrist and fingers limited by pain, discomfort, and an unwillingness to move. As this was his nondominant arm, the impact of his scholastic activities may not be as high as compared to an injury of his dominant arm.

Diagnostic Evaluations

Radiographs were obtained, anterior–posterior (AP) and lateral views (Figure 2.1). The lateral view confirmed a posterolateral dislocation of his right elbow. The distal humerus was anterior to the coronoid process of the ulna. The radius and ulna appeared to have maintained a normal relationship with each other. No fractures were evident on x-rays. Postreduction AP and lateral radiographs were taken (Figure 2.2). Because no fractures were evident on radiographs and stability was maintained through passive ROM postreduction, further advanced imaging was not warranted.

Diagnosis

Elbow dislocation.

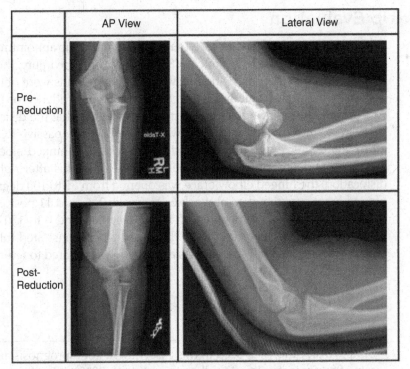

	AP View	Lateral View
Pre-Reduction		
Post-Reduction		

FIGURE 2.1 (Top) Radiographs demonstrating elbow dislocation.

FIGURE 2.2 (Bottom) Radiographs demonstrating post-reduction elbow x-rays.

Interventions

The patient underwent a conscious sedation in the ED to perform the reduction. Joint reduction is required in an urgent manner to decrease the risk of further damage to the surrounding neurovascular structures. After reduction was completed, secondary radiographs were performed to confirm congruent reduction and ensure that no fractures or incarcerated fragments were seen within the joint. The patient was then placed in a posterior fiberglass splint in approximately 90 degrees of elbow flexion with the forearm in neutral as the elbow was stable through a full passive ROM following reduction. He was instructed to follow up in 1 week following reduction at the sports medicine/orthopedic clinic.

Patient Education

Educate the patient and the family about the importance of physical therapy and working on gradually increasing ROM and restoring strength. Instruct the patient to remain in the brace at all times except during physical therapy appointments.

Follow-Up Evaluation

Continuation of treatment included subsequent follow-up appointment at an outpatient sports medicine clinic. At 8 days following the injury, the patient reported improvement in pain and swelling. Radiographs were obtained to confirm a maintained elbow joint reduction and no evidence of fractures. At this time the splint was removed in order to assess that the distal neurovascular exam remained intact. He was able to tolerate passive ROM from 60 to 100 degrees without pain, and was placed in a hinged elbow brace locked at 90 degrees for 1 more week. At 2 weeks status after right elbow dislocation, the hinged elbow brace was opened from 75 to 100 degrees. The hinged brace was removed at week 6. At weeks 2, 6, and 11 postreduction, his ROM was 30 to 110 degrees, 10 to 130 degrees, and 0 to 130 degrees, respectively. At 11 weeks following the injury he demonstrated full, stable, pain-free ROM, and full strength. As a result, he was cleared to return to full, unrestricted sports participation.

CLINICAL PEARL

Simple dislocations, as seen in this case, have a good prognosis and low rate of future instability (Middleton & Anakwe, 2012). It has been shown in the literature for simple elbow dislocations that early active ROM while maintaining joint stability in the rehabilitation program is crucial in predicting better long-term outcomes (Armstrong, 2015).

REFERENCES

Adirim, T. A., & Cheng, T. L. (2003). Overview of injuries in the young athlete. *Sports Medicine, 33*(1), 75.

Armstrong, A. (2015). Simple elbow dislocation. *Hand Clinics, 31,* 521–531.

Dizdarevic, I., Low, S., Currie, D. W., Comstock, R. D., Hammoud, S., & Atanda, A. (2016). Epidemiology of elbow dislocations in high school athletes. *American Journal of Sports Medicine, 44*(1), 202–208.

Middleton, S. D., & Anakwe, R. E. (2012). Focus on elbow dislocation. *Journal of Bone & Joint Surgery.*

Stoneback, J. W., Owens, B. D., Sykes, J., Athwal, G. S., Pointer, L., & Wolf, J. (2012). Incidence of elbow dislocations in the United States population. *Journal of Bone & Joint Surgery, American, 94-A*(3), 240–245.

Case Study 2.2: Acute Nursemaid's Elbow (annular ligament displacement)

Kimberly A. Joerg

SETTING: ORTHOPEDIC URGENT CARE

Definition and Incidence

Nursemaid's elbow or annular ligament displacement was formerly termed "radial head subluxation." Most commonly, the injury is seen in children between ages 1 and 4, and occurs when there is a sudden forceful traction on the hand when the forearm is pronated and the elbow is extended (Browner, 2013).

Patient

A 3-year-old girl presents with her mother. The mother states, "My daughter has not been using her left arm since this afternoon." According to the mother, earlier this afternoon the father was helping child put on her coat and pulled child's arm through sleeve. Since then, parents have noticed that she has not been using left arm and continues to hold it very still. Otherwise the child is healthy, no prior hospitalizations or surgeries, is up to date with immunizations, and has no known allergies. She is not using the left arm, but is using all other extremities per parents; no rashes; denies numbness or tingling.

Physical Assessment

The child is sitting on mother's lap guarding left arm and holding it still against her body. She is not actively moving or using it, even when prompted with a sticker. There is no swelling, redness, or bruising noted of left arm. On palpation, there is mild tenderness at left radial head. The bilateral upper extremities are warm, pink, brisk capillary refill, positive radial pulse, positive sensation, positive motion noted of right upper extremity. However, there is minimal movement of left arm and fingers of left hand.

Diagnostic Evaluations

Standard of care recommends that radiographs of elbow are not necessary unless after two attempts to reduce, the elbow does not return to baseline or there is suspicion of a fracture (Browner, 2013). Ultrasound and MRI may also be utilized if history is not clear, two attempts at reduction are not effective, or if injury or tear to ligament is suspected (Wolfman, 2015).

Diagnosis

Nursemaid's elbow, annular ligament displacement.

Interventions

The child was kept in the parent's lap, the child's left elbow was held in the provider's hand. With the provider's other hand, the left forearm was pronated then fully extended, no "click" was felt by the provider after the attempt. After observing the child for 30 minutes, there was limited movement of the left arm. The procedure was repeated using more traction and a "click" was felt (Browner, 2013). After the second attempt of the pronation technique, the child was observed using and moving the left arm without difficulty within 30 minutes. She reached for a popsicle and was able to bring it to her mouth with her left arm. Her parents were educated about incidence of reoccurrence (up to one third) and to avoid tugging motion to the arms (Browner, 2013). The child was discharged without any restrictions.

Patient Education

It is important to educate the family on the mechanism of injury for annular ligament displacements (nursemaid's elbow), and how to prevent future incidents.

Follow-Up Evaluation

Generally, no follow-up is necessary for this injury. It is good practice to educate the family and to avoid future incidents. Provide information to the family to seek follow-up if the child is demonstrating any unexpected changes in use of the arm, pain, numbness, or any concerning symptoms.

REFERENCES

Browner, E. (2013). Brief: Nursemaid's elbow (annular ligament displacement). *Pediatrics in Review, 34*(8), 366–367.
Wolfram, W. (2015). Nursemaid elbow. Retrieved from http://emedicine.medscape.com/article/803026-overview

Case Study 2.3: Acute Olecranon Bursitis

Karen M. Myrick

SETTING: URGENT CARE

Definition and Incidence

The olecranon bursa is protective of friction. The olecranon bursa is susceptible to pressure, trauma, infection, and inflammatory conditions because of its subcutaneous and anatomical position (Sayegh & Strauch, 2014). Bursitis is inflammation of the bursa, and can result from one or a number of causes.

Patient

Patient presents with the chief complaint of right elbow discomfort and swelling after slipping on the ice and striking his elbow yesterday. Swelling occurred within a couple of hours of the injury, and has formed a rather round and full area over his elbow. He denies any fever, chills or malaise, and had not had similar symptoms in the past. Discomfort is well located in the left elbow, and very mild in nature. Swelling is concerning to the patient and his mother, with whom he presents. He denies any loss of motion, and did try to ice for 20 minutes twice yesterday, which did not alleviate the swelling. He tried ibuprofen, 800 mg at bedtime last night, but the swelling was unchanged upon awakening. He denies any numbness, tingling, or paresthesias.

Social History

This 21-year-old male is in his junior year of college, and plays intercollegiate hockey. He lives at school, 1.5 hours away from home.

CLINICAL PEARL

Given the history of trauma in this case, the likelihood of other causative factors is decreased. The nurse practitioner must rule out the differential diagnosis of infection, crystal-induced arthropathy, prolonged pressure, and inflammatory arthritis.

Physical Assessment

The patient is a 21-year-old male who is in no acute distress. He has no discomfort throughout the physical examination. He is 6′0″ and weighs 191 lb. On inspection, there is a moderate sized swelling over the olecranon bursa. The swelling is well contained in a round shape. There is no erythema or lymphangitis noted, no open cuts or abrasions. With palpation, the moderate area of swelling is palpable, and no joint effusion is appreciated. ROM in the elbow is full from −5 of extension to 135 degrees of flexion and 90 degrees of pronation and supination. He describes a feeling of "tightness" and "stiffness" with full flexion. Biceps and triceps strength testing is 5/5 and equal to the contralateral side. There are no focal neurological deficits in the right upper extremity.

Diagnostic Evaluations

A radiograph was obtained, and did not demonstrate a fracture of dislocation in a skeletally mature male.

Diagnosis

Olecranon bursitis.

Interventions

The patient was placed in to a compression dressing with an elbow pad, and told to limit the pressure on the elbow and over use of the arm. He was encouraged to leave the compressive dressing in place and return in 2 weeks for follow-up.

Patient Education

Encourage the patient to keep the dressing on, because the compression is typically very helpful in eliminating the swelling of the bursa (Baumbach, Lobo, Badyine, Mutschler, & Kanz, 2014). Encourage patience with the resolution of symptoms, as olecranon bursitis typically will resolve without invasive intervention. Although many patients will want to have the bursa drained, the possibility of developing infection of complications is high, and the treatment algorithm should begin with the least invasive options.

Follow-Up Evaluation

Follow-up after the 2-week time period revealed decreased swelling in the olecranon bursa, increased patient discomfort, and full ROM. At this time, the patient was encouraged to continue to wear the compressive dressing for the next 1 to 2 weeks, and to return if swelling continued beyond that time.

REFERENCES

Baumbach, S., Lobo, C., Badyine, I., Mutschler, W., & Kanz, K. (2014). Prepatellar and olecranon bursitis: Literature review and development of a treatment algorithm. *Archives of Orthopaedic & Trauma Surgery, 134*(3), 359–370.

Sayegh, E., & Strauch, R. (2014). Treatment of olecranon bursitis: A systematic review. *Archives of Orthopaedic & Trauma Surgery, 134*(11), 1517–1536.

Case Study 2.4: Chronic Lateral Epicondylitis

Scott A. Myrick

SETTING: PRIMARY CARE

Definition and Incidence

Lateral epicondylitis is a common cause of elbow pain (Soyoung, Youngjun, & Wanhee, 2014). Athletes participating in such overhead sports as tennis and baseball are exposed to a higher likelihood of injury from the repetitive nature of their activity. Seldom do tennis players, for example, expose their dominant arm to periods of relative rest during practice or a match, save for the occasional two-handed strike.

Forces across tendons can cause micro trauma that manifests itself initially as intermittent pain, which can develop into the inability to grip a racket. This can lead to difficulty in performing simple tasks not related to sports.

Patient

A 20-year-old female tennis player in her junior year at a local university presents with right elbow pain that has been present for the last month, and is worse with activity, and better with rest. Pain is a 7 out of 10 with grasping, and 2 out of 10 at rest. She is a good-natured woman very passionate about her sport. She is competitive in nature and is preparing for the upcoming season of outdoor tennis, having just completed an indoor camp that ran for 6 weeks. The patient provides a history of recently attempting new techniques her coach said would help with her striking power, and has a new tennis racket with a larger grip, another recommendation of her coach. She is very active in social activities at her school but admits that her chief activity is tennis. She's been playing since she was 8 years old and does take it quite seriously.

Social History

The patient has been playing tennis for 12 years and, after her college career ends, hopes to continue this play at the recreational level. She does admit to playing tennis year round despite being advised to rest. She does not drink or smoke and, outside tennis, does participate in a strength and conditioning program authored by her coach. She has an aggressive course load in her third year and uses tennis as an outlet for any stress she encounters with school. At the end of her semester, she plans to do a semester abroad where she hopes to be exposed to a different level of tennis.

CLINICAL PEARL
For those participating in overhead sports, regular rest is important to prevent overuse injuries. The ability to add strength training and increase or maintain flexibility can contribute greatly to a healthy season and enhanced performance.

Physical Assessment

Presentation of the patient shows no acute distress. She is 5'6" and weighs 140 lb. Upon examination of the affected elbow, there is no visible swelling apparent. Palpation of the elbow medially reveals no soreness. However, on the lateral side just distal to the lateral epicondyle, quite exquisite tenderness is elicited. Sensation generally in the arm distal to the elbow is normal and there are no other signs of neurological deficits. ROM is full, −5 degrees extension and full flexion to 135 degrees. These motions passively do not cause specific pain. With resisted flexion, the patient complains of no discomfort but does have some pain with resisted extension. Supination and pronation also cause no immediate pain, nor does resisted wrist flexion. Upon resisted wrist extension, however, the pain that brings the patient to the office is elicited. This pain is particularly pronounced with resisted extension of not only the wrist in general but more so with resisted extension of the middle phalanx. Testing of strength is normal, 5/5. With ligamentous testing of the elbow, both varus and valgus stress testing is normal both at 0 and 30 degrees of elbow flexion.

Diagnostic Evaluations

Due to the patient's high activity level, a radiograph was obtained to look for the presence of any avulsion or bony fragments. Radiographs were negative. A MRI was obtained. The MRI demonstrated obvious inflammation surrounding the lateral epicondyle.

Diagnosis

Lateral epicondylitis of the right elbow.

Interventions

The patient was educated on resting her arm from aggravating movements including gripping, on not playing tennis, and on applying ice four to six times daily. She was also instructed on a regimen of nonsteroidal anti-inflammatory drugs (NSAIDs) to be taken daily with food; 800 mg of ibuprofen was ordered. A routine of physical therapy was prescribed for two to three times a week for 6 weeks, with a focus on strengthening the musculature both proximal and distal to the elbow joint as well as postural muscles surrounding the shoulder joint. Vigorous stretching of the extensor group of muscles on the posterior forearm along with friction massage was also suggested.

Patient Education

Educate the patient about how changes to a training regime, practice routine, or equipment can have an effect on their soft tissues, including tendons. Seemingly simple changes such as changing a grip, attempting a new technique, or changes in the training regimen can cause dramatic changes physiologically.

When changes are implemented, recommend changing one thing at a time, so as not to confuse the causative factor if something ends in discomfort or injury. While training etiquette is paramount, it is also important to educate the patient to avoid aggravating activity, especially repetitive maneuvers and throwing. The potential for further aggravation is high and could lead to a much longer recovery time. Teach the patient that most cases resolve in time, and emphasize the need for rest from the causative motion, evaluation of the overhead mechanics, and a graduated return to activity.

Follow-Up Evaluation

Follow-up at 6 weeks was arranged to gauge progress, and demonstrated that she was having minimal discomfort, and working on a home exercise program and gradual return-to-play program. Typically nonoperative, lateral epicondylitis or "tennis elbow" can resolve with rest and therapy, but corticosteroid injections and surgical intervention can also be used in persistent cases.

REFERENCE

Soyoung, L., Youngjun, K., & Wanhee, L. (2014). Changes in pain, dysfunction, and grip strength of patients with acute lateral epicondylitis caused by frequency of physical therapy: A randomized controlled trial. *Journal of Physical Therapy Science, 26*(7), 1037–1040. doi:10.1589/jpts.26.1037

Case Study 2.5: Chronic Cubital Tunnel Syndrome

Karen M. Myrick

SETTING: PRIMARY CARE

Definition and Incidence

Secondary only to carpal tunnel syndrome, cubital tunnel syndrome is the second most common nerve compression in the upper extremity (Kroonen, 2012).

Patient

A 33-year-old woman presents to the clinic with the complaint of right hand numbness and tingling, mostly in the fourth and fifth fingers. The symptoms have been bothering her for the past 3 months, and are present when she has a long conversation on the phone, and also awakens her at night four or five nights a week. There is no pain, she states, but the numbness and tingling is bothersome.

Social History

She is a nurse on the labor and delivery unit of the hospital. She is active with swimming and bicycling. She does not have any children and is single.

> **CLINICAL PEARL**
>
> It is important to rule out the neck as the cause of numbness and tingling in the hand. In the case of the fourth and fifth fingers, a problem with the nerve routes at C7, C8, and T1 should be included in the differential diagnosis list.

Physical Assessment

On inspection, there is no muscle wasting appreciated; no scars or evidence of trauma. The interossei and hypothenar eminence are equal in bulk and strength to the left, unaffected arm. Palpation reveals no masses or swelling over the ulnar nerve root, and no subluxation of the nerve is appreciated. Sensation is intact to sharp and light touch in all three ulnar sensory areas of the hand (digital branch, palmar cutaneous nerve, and dorsal cutaneous nerve). ROM is from −5 to 135 degrees in the elbow. A Tinel test at the elbow is positive, as is a flexion test. A Spurling's maneuver is negative, as is any motion of the neck for reproduction of symptoms.

CLINICAL PEARL

Tinel testing is performed by percussion over the ulnar nerve in the ulnar groove, and cubital tunnel. The flexion test is maximal elbow flexion sustained for 1 minute or until symptoms are reproduced.

Diagnostic Evaluations

A radiograph was not obtained, due to the lack of yield on information that would be likely in this patient. An electromyography (EMG) is ordered and demonstrates mild to moderate ulnar neuropathy.

CLINICAL PEARL

EMG is useful for confirming the diagnosis, and to rule out other causes (Smith & DeSantis, 2014). EMG is also beneficial in helping to determine severity, or to document baseline results. This information is typically helpful for provider and patients as well, in determining the best treatment plan.

Diagnosis

Cubital tunnel syndrome.

Interventions

A discussion of treatment options is provided for the patient. She opts to try a pillow splint at night, and to decrease time with her elbow flexed. Follow-up is recommended for 6 weeks.

Patient Education

Educating the patient about the possibility for worsening symptoms is important. It is also important to discuss that surgical intervention may be necessary, should symptoms persist with conservative management.

Follow-Up Evaluation

On return visit, the patient noted that her symptoms were persistent, despite the activity modifications and conservative measures that were followed. She was sent for a surgical consultation at this point in time, and had an elective ulnar nerve decompression. Her symptoms resolved after surgical intervention.

REFERENCES

Kroonen, L. T. (2012). Cubital tunnel syndrome. *Orthopedic Clinics of North America, 43*(4), 475–486. doi:10.1016/j.ocl.2012.07.017

Smith, R. M., & DeSantis, A. (2014). Atypical ulnar neuropathy localized with Tinel's sign: A case report. *American Journal of Physical Medicine & Rehabilitation* (Suppl.), a17–a18.

Case Study 2.6: Little Leaguer's Elbow (medial epicondyle apophysitis)

Scott A. Myrick

SETTING: PRIMARY CARE

Definition and Incidence

Repetitive throwing causes forces across the elbow that are compressive on the lateral side and tensile on the medial joint (Shanley & Thigpen, 2013). Repetitive strain without adequate rest and muscle imbalances may lead to apophysitis (Myrick, 2015).

Younger athletes who engage in more than one overhead sport or do not get adequate rest are more prone to overuse injuries.

Patient

A 14-year-old baseball pitcher patient presents with right elbow pain. Pain is worse with throwing, and better with rest. With throwing, pain is described as an 8 out of 10, and at rest it is a 3 to 4 out of 10. He has tried ibuprofen, 600 mg once or twice without any relief. He has also tried ice in the evening a couple of times that helps while it is on. He denies any numbness or tingling, and describes his arm as feeling weak. There is no specific traumatic event that he is aware of. His current elbow pain has kept him from participating in sports for the past 2 weeks.

Social History

This 14-year-old male is an eighth grader at a local school. Outside of his school obligations, he plays often with friends and is active in multiple baseball

---

CLINICAL PEARLS

For those participating in overhead sports, regular rest is important to prevent overuse injuries. The ability to add strength training can contribute greatly to a healthy season and enhanced performance.

Pain that is worse in throwing activities and better with rest is typical in the history of the present illness for patients with medial epicondyle aphophysitis.

leagues. He is a good student who regularly is on the honor roll. Generally quiet in nature, he is a motivated athlete who wishes to return to full activity.

Physical Assessment

He is in no acute distress. He is 5'8" and weighs 151 lb. On inspection, there is no visible swelling or deformity. With palpation on the medial side of the elbow, tenderness is elicited over the medial collateral ligament (MCL). No tenderness is evident on the lateral side of the elbow. The patient does not have full extension of the elbow, which is inhibited by pain, lacking approximately 10 degrees. Passive flexion with a feeling of stiffness and pain is 120 degrees. When flexing the elbow, the endpoint is soft. Strength testing elbow flexion and extension displays good strength with some residual pain. Supination itself with a flexed elbow is sound; however, pronation elicits increased soreness over the MCL. With ligamentous testing of the elbow, both varus and valgus stress testing is normal with slight pain at 0 degrees. However, at 30 degrees of flexion, there is significant pain and an obvious gapping with a valgus force. Neurologically, the patient has no focal deficits.

Diagnostic Evaluations

A radiograph was obtained to look for the presence of any avulsion. Diagnosis is typically made with clinical examination only. However, radiographs can be helpful to demonstrate hypertrophy, widening and fragmentation of the apophysis, especially with a comparison view of the contralateral side. Figure 2.3 demonstrates widening of the medial apophysis.

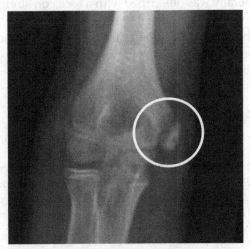

FIGURE 2.3 Radiograph demonstrating widening of the medial aphophysis of the elbow in a little leaguer.

Diagnosis

Medial epicondyle apophysitis.

Interventions

The patient and family were provided education on this condition; instructions for resting his arm from aggravating movements including absolutely no throwing, and icing four to six times daily were provided. He was also instructed on a regimen of NSAIDs to be taken daily with food; ibuprofen 600 mg three times a day.

Patient Education

Educate the patient on rest of the arm. This includes throwing other types of balls, which is often times not thought of, and the patient interprets the communication as avoiding only pitching a baseball. Explicit instructions on no throwing activity should clearly include any throwing movements, including that of snowballs.

Keeping the athlete from all throwing activities until there is no pain typically consists of a 4- to 6-week initial trial of rest. Upon completion of this rest period, a follow-up appointment is encouraged. Dependent upon the history and physical examination findings at that follow-up visit, a strength program focusing on hip, trunk, and back musculature is indicated.

Follow-Up Evaluation

At the 6-week visit, the patient was feeling less discomfort at rest; occasionally a dull ache was reported that was rated a 1 out of 10. He was very anxious to get back to his activities. A slow progression was recommended, and physical therapy was prescribed with a focus on strengthening the musculature both proximal and distal to the elbow joint as well as postural muscles surrounding the shoulder joint. Another visit was made for 6 weeks out, and at that time, the patient was progressing to a throwing program, and returning to activity pain free.

REFERENCES

Myrick, K. M. (2015). Pediatric overuse sports injury and injury prevention. *Journal for Nurse Practitioners, 11*(10), 1023–1031. doi:10.1016/j.nurpra.2015.08.028

Shanley, E., & Thigpen, C. (2013). Throwing injuries in the adolescent athlete. *International Journal of Sports Physical Therapy, 8*(5), 630–640.

CHAPTER 3

Wrist

Case Study 3.1: Acute Fracture

Hardeep Singh and Craig M. Rodner

SETTING: ORTHOPEDIC URGENT CARE OR EMERGENCY DEPARTMENT

Definition and Incidence

Wrist fractures are one of the most common orthopedic injuries presenting in two age groups: younger individuals as a result of high-energy trauma, and older individuals as a result of low-energy trauma, classically falls.

Patient

A 65-year-old female presents to the emergency department after a fall onto her right outstretched hand while jogging. She was able to get herself up; however, she had pain, swelling, and a deformity in her right wrist immediately after the fall. Pain is rated at a 9 out of 10, and worse with any movement. The patient reports that she is unable to move her wrist due to the pain and denies any numbness or tingling. The patient denies any loss of consciousness, head trauma, or other musculoskeletal injuries.

Social History

This 65-year-old woman is a retired schoolteacher, and is very active in running. She is currently training for a 10-km race that takes place in 3 months.

Physical Assessment

Upon physical examination, the patient is in mild distress due to her discomfort. Her wrist has visible swelling and deformity. The skin is intact and motor function intact in her extensor pollicis longus (radial nerve), flexor pollicis longus (median nerve), and hand intrinsic muscles (ulnar nerve). Sensation is intact in the median, ulnar, and radial nerve distributions and she has a palpable radial pulse. Elbow range of motion is full.

Diagnostic Evaluations

Radiographs are taken, and include poster anterior (PA) and lateral views of the wrist (Figure 3.1). The wrist is examined for radial inclination (normal 23 degrees), radial height (normal 11–13 mm), and volar tilt (normal 11 degrees) (Lafontaine, 1989). The x-rays reveal that the patient has a right distal radius fracture with loss of radial height, radial inclination, and volar tilt.

Diagnosis

Distal radius fracture, displaced.

Interventions

The patient is given a hematoma block, which was performed at the fracture site using 10 mL of 1% lidocaine without epinephrine to provide adequate anesthesia. The patient's arm was then subsequently hung onto an intravenous (IV) pole using finger traps to provide traction, also known as "ligamentotaxis." The fracture was reduced by recreating the mechanism of

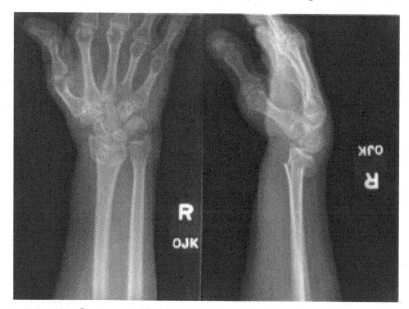

FIGURE 3.1 Poster anterior (PA) and lateral views of the right wrist demonstrating a distal radius fracture with dorsal angulation.

injury, which included hyperextending the wrist and providing longitudinal traction as used to perform a closed reduction. A sugar-tong splint was applied and molded with a three-point mold to hold the reduction. X-rays were repeated to assess the adequacy of reduction.

Patient Education

In the urgent care setting, it is important that the patient understands the need to follow up within 1 week to assess the wrist fracture and discuss management options. Patient should not bear weight on the affected extremity and should keep it elevated to help with swelling control.

Follow-Up Evaluation

Postreduction x-rays are assessed for radial inclination, radial height, and volar tilt. It is important to also evaluate the neurologic status of the extremity after reduction (Litchman, 2010). As this injury requires surgical consultation, it is possible that the nurse practitioner may not follow up directly with the patient. If the nurse practitioner is in a setting working collaboratively with an orthopedic surgeon, the nurse may perform the preoperative and postoperative care of the patient, and may be in a position to assist in the operating room. For the primary care nurse practitioner, it is likely the patient will return after surgical intervention and rehab has been completed, and the patient has been discharged from the specialist. The patient was referred in consultation with hand surgery. She decided to undergo operative treatment for her right distal radius fracture, which included an open reduction and internal fixation (ORIF) with a volar distal radius locking plate, restoring the radial height, radial inclination, and volar tilt, as shown in Figure 3.2.

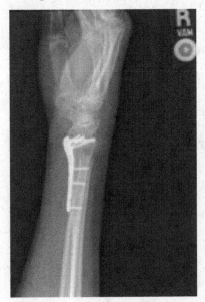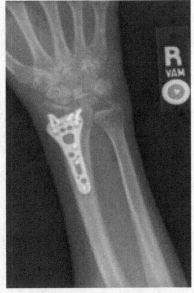

FIGURE 3.2 Posteroanterior (PA) and lateral views of the right wrist after having undergone open reduction and internal fixation with a volar plate. The radial height, radial inclination, and volar tilt are restored.

CLINICAL PEARL

Be sure to evaluate radiographs for radial height, radial inclination, and volar tilt. Acceptable parameters for an adequate reduction include: less than 5 mm of radial shortening, less than 5 degrees of change in radial inclination, less than 2-mm articular step off, and dorsal angulation of less than 5 degrees.

REFERENCES

Lafontaine, M., Hardy, D., & Delince, P. (1989). Stability assessment of distal radius fractures. *Injury, 20*(4), 208–210.

Lichtman, D. M., Randipsingh, R., Boyer, M. I., Putnam, M. D., Ring, D., Slutsky, D. J., … Raymond, L. (2010). Treatment of distal radius fractures. *Journal of the American Academy of Orthopaedic Surgeons, 18*(3), 180–189.

Case Study 3.2: Acute DeQuervain's Tenosynovitis

Hardeep Singh and Craig M. Rodner

SETTING: ACUTE VISIT IN THE ORTHOPEDIC OFFICE

Definition and Incidence

DeQuervain's disease is a common pathology of the wrist, and often results from overuse. Pain is generated from resisted gliding of the tendons (abductor pollicis longus and extensor pollicis brevis) in the first dorsal compartment of the wrist (Haque et al., 2015).

Patient

A 40-year-old female presents with an insidious onset of right radial-sided wrist pain for 2 months. The pain is localized above the radial styloid and is worse with activity. She rates the pain as a 4 out of 10 at rest, and 7 out of 10 with activity. She denies any history of trauma. She denies having tried anything to relieve her symptoms. She denies any numbness or tingling in the wrist or hand.

Social History

Patient works as a secretary and is unable to continue typing due to the pain in her wrist. She is married and lives with her husband and her 7-year-old daughter.

Physical Assessment

On physical examination, she is in no acute distress. Inspection reveals minimal swelling over the right radial styloid. With palpation, the first dorsal compartment (abductor pollicis longus and extensor pollicis brevis) is tender. She has full, nonpainful range of motion in her fingers and elbow.

Diagnostic Evaluation

A Finkelstein test is performed and found to be positive. Because the diagnosis of acute DeQuervain's tenosynovitis is a clinical diagnosis, radiographs are not necessary.

Diagnosis

DeQuervain's tenosynovitis.

> **CLINICAL PEARL**
>
> The Finkelstein test is confirmatory for DeQuervain's tenosynovitis. The Finkelstein test is performed by making a fist over the thumb and then moving the hand into ulnar deviation, which passively stretches the thumb tendons over the radial styloid (Shehab & Mirabelli, 2013). Pain with this motion is considered a positive test.

Interventions

Treatment options are discussed with the patient. The patient is given a thumb spica splint (see Figure 3.3) to rest her thumb and is given a corticosteroid injection (40-mg Depo-Mederol or Kenalog) into the first dorsal compartment. It is recommended to the patient to rest her wrist, use the thumb spica splint for comfort, and follow up in 4 weeks.

Patient Education

Importantly, teach the patient that she has options for the treatment of her condition. These treatment options range from conservative to operative in

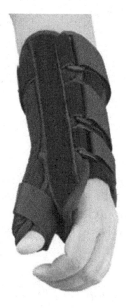

FIGURE 3.3 A thumb spica splint.

nature and are a stepwise process. Rest and modalities to decrease inflammation are the first line of treatment and include oral anti-inflammatory medications such as ibuprofen (800-mg three times a day) or Naprosyn (500-mg two times a day), and splinting. If the patient is very uncomfortable, and desires an injection, then a corticosteroid injection may be given at any time in the treatment.

CLINICAL PEARL

DeQuervain's tenosynovitis is an inflammatory condition affecting the first dorsal compartment of the hand (abductor pollicis longus and extensor pollicis brevis). The condition is more prevalent in females, and oftentimes common with new mothers picking up their children.

Follow-Up Evaluation

The patient returns to the clinic at 3 and 6 months for repeat steroid injection, but has diminishing relief from each subsequent injection. The patient returns to the clinic with worsening symptoms over the first dorsal compartment and elects to undergo operative treatment. The patient is taken to the operating room and has surgical release of the first dorsal compartment. She presents to the office 2 weeks later and reports having complete pain relief.

REFERENCES

Haque, M. M., Datta, N. K., Faisal, M. A., Islam, A., Uddin, M. J., Tarik, M. M., & Hossain, M. A. (2015). Surgical decompression of resistant cases of DeQuervain's disease. *Mymensingh Medical Journal, 24*(2), 341–345. PubMed PMID: 26007263.

Shehab, R., & Mirabelli, M. H. (2013). Evaluation and diagnosis of wrist pain: A case-based approach. *American Family Physician, 87*(8), 568–573.

Case Study 3.3: Acute Scaphoid Fracture

Hardeep Singh and Craig M. Rodner

SETTING: ORTHOPEDIC URGENT CARE

Definition and Incidence

The scaphoid is the most common fractured carpal bone with an incidence of 15% in all acute wrist injuries (Ring, Jupiter, & Herndon, 2000). The most common mechanism of injury is an axial load on a hyperextended and radially deviated wrist; common in contact sports.

Patient

A 21-year-old male presents with right wrist pain after landing on his wrist while playing rugby. He reports to have been using a splint for comfort since his injury; however, the pain has continued to progress. He denies numbness or tingling. He is unable to continue playing rugby due to his wrist pain. Pain is a 4 out of 10 at rest, and an 8 out of 10 with activity involving the wrist.

Social History

The patient is a 21-year-old college junior who plays rugby at a Division 2 school. He is studying biology, and is right-hand dominant.

Physical Assessment

Upon physical examination, the patient is in no acute distress. There is mild swelling on inspection, and there are no obvious bony abnormalities or soft-tissue changes. There is pain and tenderness upon palpation of the anatomic snuffbox. There is no pain or tenderness upon palpation of the rest of his hand. He is distally neurovascularly intact.

CLINICAL PEARL

Pain at the anatomic snuffbox is indicative of scaphoid fracture. The anatomic snuffbox is the triangular area of depression on the radial aspect of the wrist. The medial border is formed by tendon of extensor pollicis longus and the lateral border is formed by tendon of abductor pollicis longus and extensor pollicis brevis. The floor is formed by the scaphoid and trapezium.

Diagnostic Evaluations

X-rays of the left wrist are obtained (PA, lateral, and scaphoid view of wrist). A minimally displaced fracture of the waist of the scaphoid is seen (Figure 3.4). A computerized tomography (CT) scan is sometimes helpful in evaluating the location of the fracture, its size, displacement, and presence of nonunion or union. MRI is the most sensitive imaging modality for diagnosis of occult fracture within 24 hours.

Fracture can occur in three locations: Proximal pole (highest risk of nonunion, due to retrograde blood supply of the scaphoid bone); the waist (most common); and the distal pole of scaphoid.

Diagnosis

Scaphoid fracture.

Interventions

The patient is given a thumb spica cast with the interphalangeal joint free and asked to refrain from athletic activity. He undergoes a CT scan of the left wrist to further define the fracture at the proximal pole of the scaphoid (Figure 3.5).

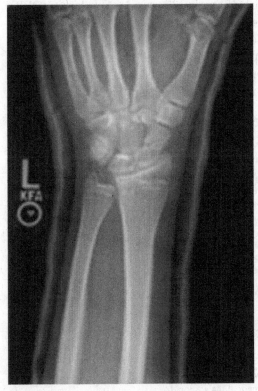 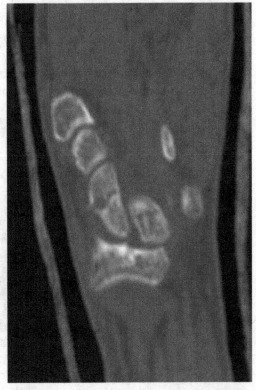

FIGURE 3.4 Posteroanterior (PA) x-ray of the left radius demonstrating a minimally displaced fracture of the scaphoid.

FIGURE 3.5 CT scan of the left wrist defining the minimally displaced fracture of the scaphoid.

CLINICAL PEARLS

Failure to diagnose and treat a scaphoid fracture may lead to nonunion, which can further lead to scaphoid nonunion advanced collapse (SNAC) (Trumble, 2003). Major blood supply to scaphoid is from the dorsal carpal branch of the radial artery supplying proximal 80% of scaphoid with retrograde blood supply. The superficial palmar arch enters the distal tubercle supplying the distal 20% of the scaphoid.

Advanced collapse and progressive arthritis of the wrist starting at the radial styloid and scaphoid, progressing to the scaphocapitate arthrosis and to the periscaphoid arthrosis, eventually leads to dorsal intercalated segment instability of the wrist (Gutow, 2007).

Patient Education

Educate the patient on the possibility of a nonunion of the scaphoid, and the physiology behind the reasoning.

Follow-Up Evaluation

After referral to the orthopedic surgeon, this patient elects to undergo operative treatment to decrease the risk of scaphoid nonunion. He has an ORIF. He is immobilized in a thumb spica splint postoperatively. The patient is asked to remain in his thumb spica splint postoperatively and be nonweight bearing. He is asked to follow up in clinic in 1 week to evaluate how he is doing. Short-term narcotics are prescribed for pain control. Repeat x-rays are taken when the patient presents for postoperative visit (Figure 3.6).

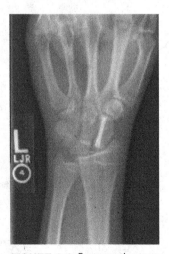

FIGURE 3.6 Postoperative x-ray of the left wrist, following operative treatment of the scaphoid fracture.

REFERENCES

Gutow, A. P. (2007). Percutaneous fixation of scaphoid fractures. *Journal of the American Academy of Orthopaedic Surgeons, 15*(8), 474–485.

Ring, D., Jupiter, J. B., & Herndon, J. H. (2000). Acute fractures of the scaphoid. *Journal of the American Academy of Orthopaedic Surgeons, 8*(4), 225–231.

Trumble, T. E. (2003). Management of scaphoid nonunions. *Journal of the American Academy of Orthopaedic Surgeons, 11*(6), 380–391.

Case Study 3.4: Chronic Carpal Tunnel Syndrome

Hardeep Singh and Craig M. Rodner

SETTING: OUTPATIENT HAND CLINIC

Definition and Incidence

Carpal tunnel syndrome is the most common entrapment neuropathy of the upper extremity, as a result of compression of the median nerve in the carpal tunnel (De Krom et al., 1992). The most common cause of carpal tunnel is inflamed synovium. Acute carpal tunnel syndrome can be a complication of a distal radius fracture or a perilunate dislocation (Keith et al., 2009).

Patient

The patient is a 55-year-old female presenting to the hand clinic for 4 months of progressively worsening right-hand numbness and tingling in the thumb, index, middle, and half the ring fingers. She reports the numbness is intermittent, worse at night to the point where she wakes up and has to shake the feeling off her hands. She states that she feels a little weaker in her right hand and has difficulty opening jars now. She denies any recent trauma, denies any neck pain radiating down. The numbness and tingling are localized in the radial three digits and are isolated to her hand.

Social History

This 55-year-old woman is the owner of a dance studio, where she manages the class schedule, website, registrations, and recitals. She has three children, all living nearby, and one grandchild on the way.

Physical Assessment

Physical examination reveals a pleasant female in no acute distress. On inspection, there is no atrophy of her thenar muscles. Sensation is decreased in the radial 3.5 digits. She has a positive Durkan's compression test (compression of the carpal tunnel for 60 seconds), Tinel's sign (percussion on the median nerve), and Phalen's sign (wrist flexion for 60 seconds). She has full range of motion of her neck, without any elicitation of symptoms, and a negative Spurling's maneuver.

Diagnostic Evaluations

X-rays are not needed in the clinical diagnosis of carpal tunnel; however, it may be helpful to rule out bone pathology as the cause of the patient's pain. An MRI or ultrasound of the wrist is useful when a mass is suspected as the cause of acute carpal tunnel syndrome, which is rare.

Electrodiagnostic studies, electromyogram and nerve conduction velocity (EMG/NCV), are the gold standard in diagnosis of chronic carpal tunnel syndrome (Keith et al., 2009). They can reveal NCV slowing without fibrillations and sharp waves in thenar muscles, which can be seen in more advanced cases with motor involvement.

Diagnosis

Carpal tunnel syndrome.

Interventions

Given her clinical history and physical examination findings she is diagnosed with chronic carpal tunnel syndrome. She is given a wrist splint to wear at night and a corticosteroid injection (40-mg Depo-Medrol or Kenalog) into the carpal tunnel to help decrease the inflammation. She returns to the clinic in 1 month reporting that she had complete relief from the injection for 2 weeks; however, the numbness and tingling have returned. She elects to undergo operative treatment to decompress the carpal tunnel.

CLINICAL PEARL

Carpal tunnel syndrome is usually a chronic condition, which presents in the clinic. Symptoms may vary from patient to patient; however, key symptoms typically include numbness/tingling specifically at night, waking the person up from sleep. Objective evaluation includes obtaining nerve conduction studies. Nonoperative treatment includes night splints, corticosteroid injections; however, operative treatment is recommended to limit damage to the median nerve.

Patient Education

It is important to educate the patient about the continuum of treatment from conservative to operative. It is equally important to discuss progression of the syndrome and the possibility for median nerve damage that is progressive and may not be reparable.

Follow-Up Evaluation

The patient decides that operative management is the best plan of care for her. She is referred to the surgeon and then follows up with the nurse practitioner. Postoperatively, the patient is asked to keep her dressing on until follow-up in the clinic. It is recommended that she not do any heavy lifting and let her wrist rest. She is asked to return to the office for postoperative evaluation 1 week after her surgery. The patient is followed closely postoperatively, and reports doing well with good pain control and remains neurovascularly intact. Her numbness and tingling have resolved and she is not waking up at night any more with numbness and tingling.

REFERENCES

De Krom, M. C., Knipschild, P. G., Kester, A. D., Thijs, C. T., Boekkooi, P. F., & Spaans, F. (1992). Carpal tunnel syndrome: Prevalence in the general population. *Journal of Clinical Epidemiology, 45*(4), 373–376.

Keith, M. W., Masear, V., Chung, K., Maupin, K., Andary, M., Amadio, P. C., . . . Wies, J. L. (2009). Diagnosis of carpal tunnel syndrome. *Journal of the American Academy of Orthopaedic Surgeons, 17*(6), 389–405.

Case Study 3.5: Ganglion Cyst

Hardeep Singh and Craig M. Rodner

SETTING: OUTPATIENT CLINIC

Definition and Incidence

Ganglion cysts are the most common hand mass, and more common on dorsal than volar aspect (Kerrigan, Bertoni, & Jaeger, 1988; Plate, Lee, Steiner, & Steiner, 2003). A ganglion is an insidious onset of swelling on dorsal or radial aspect of the wrist, and may occur as a result of trauma, mucoid degeneration, or synovial herniation. The cyst is filled with fluid from tendon sheath or joint and has no epithelial lining.

Patient

A 23-year-old presents with an insidious onset of swelling on dorsal aspect of her right wrist that began 2 months ago. She reports to have been involved in a motor vehicle crash 2 months ago but denies any injuries. The swelling is not painful and does not affect her day-to-day activities, but the cosmetic appearance bothers her. She denies any numbness, tingling, or sensation loss. She has not tried much to make it better, except for a compressive bandage, which did not help.

Social History

This 23-year-old female is the receptionist at a car dealership. She is single, and lives with her boyfriend of 2 years.

Physical Assessment

Physical examination reveals a palpable mass on the dorsal aspect of the right wrist measuring 2 cm × 2 cm. The mass is well circumscribed, firm, movable, and trans-illuminates under light. She has full range of motion and normal sensation in her wrist and hand.

CLINICAL PEARL

Typically, ganglion cysts are painless; however, they can compress a sensory nerve leading to pain.

Diagnostic Evaluations

Radiographic evaluation with x-rays is normal, and does not reveal any fractures or dislocations. The diagnosis of a ganglion cyst is a clinical diagnosis and does not warrant any further imaging.

Diagnosis

Ganglion cyst, right wrist.

Interventions

It is recommended to the patient that she may try conservative management for the ganglion cyst with simple observation. The patient elects to have aspiration of the cyst. She tolerates the procedure well.

Patient Education

Educate your patient that conservative measures may include doing nothing, compression, and aspiration; but if there is discomfort or the symptoms are intolerable, then surgical excision may be an option.

Follow-Up Evaluation

Patient follows up in 6 weeks, and is doing well at this point in time with no further discomfort.

REFERENCES

Kerrigan, J. J., Bertoni, J. M., & Jaeger, S. H. (1988). Ganglion cysts and carpal tunnel syndrome. *Journal of Hand Surgery, 13*(5), 763–765.

Plate, A. M., Lee, S. J., Steiner, G., & Posner, M. A. (2003). Tumorlike lesions and benign tumors of the hand and wrist. *Journal of the American Academy of Orthopaedic Surgeons, 11*(2), 129–141.

Case Study 3.6: Chronic Ulnar Positive Wrist

Hardeep Singh and Craig M. Rodner

SETTING: PRIMARY CARE CLINIC

Definition and Incidence

The term and finding of ulnar positive variance refer to the ulna being longer than the radius, leading to impaction of the ulna into the carpus (Shariatzadeh, 2015).

This variation in anatomy may lead to wrist pain that is caused by ulnar abutment syndrome, arthrosis, triangular fibrocartilage complex tear, and lunotriquetral tears.

In an ulnar positive variance, the ulna bears 40% of the load versus 20% of the load in a normal neutral wrist (Shariatzadeh, 2015). This is more common in females than males.

Patient

A 60-year-old female presents with ulnar-sided wrist pain for 3 to 4 months. She states she was shoveling snow when the pain started. She denies any falls or traumatic injuries to her wrist. The pain is not associated with any numbness or tingling and is worse with her daily activities. The patient is unable to do basic activities of daily living without pain such as cooking, driving, or cleaning. Pain is a 6 out of 10 most days, but with some activities it escalates to a 9 out of 10.

Social History

Patient is a college professor who is starting a phased retirement. She will have the next 6 months off.

Physical Assessment

Physical examination reveals a pleasant female in no acute distress. On evaluation, there are no skin or soft-tissue abnormalities, and no deformity. Palpation reveals tenderness along the ulna styloid, pain exacerbated with ulnar deviation, axial loading, and hypersupination of the forearm. She is distally neurovascularly intact. She has full range of motion of her wrist.

Diagnostic Evaluations

Radiographs are taken (Figure 3.7.1). The patient's ulnar variance measures 2-mm positive.

Diagnosis

Ulnar positive wrist and wrist pain.

CLINICAL PEARLS

If you are suspecting ulnar variance, communicate this with the x-ray technician. To best assess this finding, the radiograph should be taken with shoulder abducted to 90 degrees, elbow flexed to 90 degrees, and forearm in neutral rotation to accurately assess the ulnar variance.

The best way to evaluate the radiograph is to calculate the distance between a line drawn tangential to articular surface of the ulna and another drawn tangential to the lunate fossa of the radius.

Interventions

The patient is provided with both conservative and surgical options for the management of her wrist. Conservative options include symptomatic treatments to provide pain relief with the use of nonsteroidal anti-inflammatory drugs (NSAIDs) and wrist cock-up splints. She initially elects NSAIDs (ibuprofen 800 mg with food three times a day), and returns for evaluation at 4 weeks.

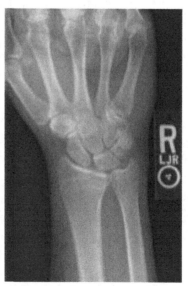

FIGURE 3.7.1 Posteroanterior (PA) of the right wrist demonstrating 2 mm of ulnar positive variance.

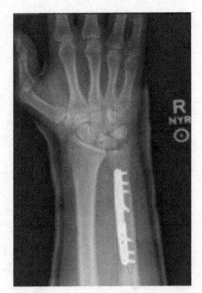

FIGURE 3.7.2 Posteroanterior (PA) of the right wrist demonstrating postoperative ulnar shortening of the ulna.

CLINICAL PEARL

Ulnar abutment syndrome results in alteration of joint forces leading to painful overload of the ulnocarpal joint, thereby causing ulnar-sided wrist pain (Tomaino & Elfar, 2005).

Patient Education

The patient is instructed to use NSAIDs and wrist cock-up splint to help improve her wrist pain. It is recommended that she rest her wrist and follow up in a month to reevaluate her pain.

Follow-Up Evaluation

When she returns, she continues to have discomfort, despite the conservative management. At this visit, she decides to undergo corticosteroid injection (40-mg Depo-Medrol or Kenalog). She has good immediate relief, and calls to schedule a follow-up visit in 9 weeks. At this point, she is referred to the orthopedic surgeon because of failed conservative management, and her continuing to have pain which is worsening. She elects to undergo ulnar-shortening osteotomy and is pain free postoperatively (Figure 3.7.2).

REFERENCES

Shariatzadeh, H. (2015). Ulnar abutment syndrome. *Shafa Orthopedic Journal, 2*(3).

Tomaino, M. M., & Elfar, J. (2005). Ulnar impaction syndrome. *Hand Clinics, 21*(4), 567–575.

CHAPTER 4

Hand

Case Study 4.1: Acute Mallet Finger

Hardeep Singh and Craig M. Rodner

SETTING: ORTHOPEDIC URGENT CARE

Definition and Incidence

A mallet finger is an acute traumatic injury resulting from a hyperflexion injury to the distal portion of the finger, the distal interphalangeal (DIP) joint resulting in forced DIP flexion (Bendre, Hartigan, & Kalainov, 2005). This type of injury leads to disruption of the terminal extensor tendon.

Patient

The patient is a 22-year-old male who presents to the emergency department after having sustained an injury to his middle finger while playing football. He reported immediate pain and swelling distally in his middle finger and inability to extend his DIP joint. He was unable to return to playing football due to the deformity of his middle finger and pain. The team athletic trainer at the game saw him, and a foam splint was put in place. It was recommended that he follow up after the game at the urgent care clinic. He denies significant pain, but has a mild ache that he rates as 4 out of 10. He is concerned about the inability to extend his finger on his own.

Social History

This 22-year-old is in his final year of college, playing at a local Division 3 university. He is single, and lives on campus. He is not working at present.

Physical Assessment

Physical examination reveals a young man who presents with his father. He is in no acute distress, but does have mild discomfort. On inspection, he had swelling and deformity of his DIP joint, with the fingertip resting in flexion. He was unable to actively extend the DIP joint. His sensation is intact, and he has no other associated symptoms.

Diagnostic Evaluations

Radiographs of his hand revealed no fracture or joint subluxation. Given the clinical history and physical examination findings, the patient suffered an acute nonbony mallet finger injury. Disruption of the terminal extensor tendon leads to the DIP joint lag clinically.

Diagnosis

Mallet finger (disruption of the terminal extensor tendon).

Interventions

The patient is placed in an extension splint of the DIP joint with proximal interphalangeal (PIP) joint free for 6 weeks around the clock.

CLINICAL PEARLS

Immediate intervention with an extension splint or operative treatment of a bony avulsion is important in restoring function and decreasing pain (Kalainov, Hoepfner, Hartigan, Carroll, & Genuario, 2005). Figure 4.1 is an example of a bony mallet.

It is important for the nurse practitioner to realize that operative treatment is indicated in patients with a bony avulsion fracture that has significant articular surface involvement and a subluxed DIP joint.

Patient Education

Instruct the patient to keep the extension splint on at all times and to rest his affected hand. Importantly, teach the patient that this includes in the shower, and while changing the splint or tape. The consequence of this position must be emphasized to your patient for a good outcome. Ask the patient to return to clinic in 6 weeks to be reevaluated and to refrain from athletic activity to prevent further injury.

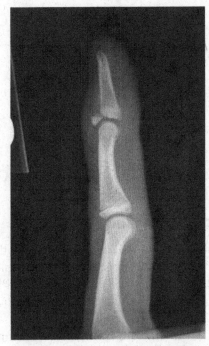

FIGURE 4.1 Radiographic example of a bony mallet.

Follow-Up Evaluation

He is seen back in the hand clinic in 6 weeks and the extension splint is removed. Physical therapy is recommended to help improve motion at the DIP joint.

REFERENCES

Bendre, A. A., Hartigan, B. J., & Kalainov, D. M. (2005). Mallet finger. *Journal of the American Academy of Orthopaedic Surgeons, 13*(5), 336–344.

Kalainov, D. M., Hoepfner, P. E., Hartigan, B. J., Carroll, C., & Genuario J. (2005). Nonsurgical treatment of closed mallet finger fractures. *Journal of Hand Surgery, 30*(3), 580–586.

Case Study 4.2: Acute Dislocation Interphalangeal Joint

Hardeep Singh and Craig M. Rodner

SETTING: ORTHOPEDIC URGENT CARE

Definition and Incidence

Dislocations of the DIP joint are typically the result of a traumatic injury to the PIP or DIP. The direction of these dislocations can be dorsal or volar, depending on the force exerted. Dorsal PIP dislocation is more common than volar dislocation and can lead to injury to the volar plate (Leggit & Meko, 2006).

Dorsal PIP fracture-dislocation—fracture is commonly located on the volar lip of the middle phalanx, with fractures involving more than 50% of the articular surface being unstable and requiring surgical treatment (Bindra & Foster, 2009). Volar PIP dislocation and fracture-dislocations are less common than dorsal dislocation, and these can lead to injury to the central slip resulting in a Boutonniere deformity.

Patient

A 20-year-old male presents with an obvious middle finger deformity after falling off his bike onto his hand. He is unable to extend or flex his middle finger at the PIP joint. He denies any numbness or tingling. He has pain that is 8 out of 10, and he is concerned over the appearance of his finger.

Social History

The patient is a 20-year-old college student. He is active socially, but does not participate in organized sports. He lives at school 2 hours away from his family.

Physical Assessment

Physical examination reveals a young man in no acute distress, but discomfort. He presents with his friend. On inspection, he has deformity of his middle finger PIP with inability to flex or extend his PIP joint. There are no soft-tissue abnormalities or open cuts, but there is a lot of dirt and mud on his hand, arms, and legs. With palpation, the middle finger is tender to palpation. There is no tenderness to palpation of his wrist, carpus, or metacarpals.

He remains neurovascularly intact; sensation is full to the finger aforementioned and following the noted deformity.

Diagnostic Evaluations

Radiographs of his hand are obtained and the lateral x-rays reveal a dorsal PIP fracture dislocation, with a volar plate avulsion fracture of the medial phalanx (Figure 4.2).

Diagnosis

Dorsal PIP fracture dislocation.

Interventions

The patient undergoes a closed reduction of his PIP with longitudinal traction and is placed in a dorsal block splint. Immediate range of motion (ROM) is started and he is asked to follow up in 1 week, at which time follow-up x-rays are obtained (Figure 4.3).

Patient Education

It is important to explain the procedure of the closed reduction to the patient quickly, and to tell the patient that most of the discomfort he will experience is while the finger is, in fact, dislocated. While reducing the dislocation with

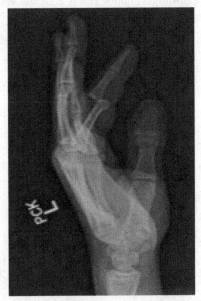

FIGURE 4.2 Radiograph of the lateral view of the hand showing a dorsal proximal interphalangeal dislocation.

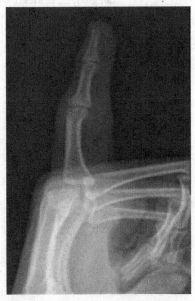

FIGURE 4.3 Post-reduction radiograph of the lateral view of the hand showing the reduced dorsal proximal interphalangeal dislocation, with joint congruity.

longitudinal traction and reproduction of the mechanism of injury will cause brief discomfort, there is usually quite a reduction in the discomfort after it is completed.

CLINICAL PEARLS

Dislocations can be simple or complex in nature. In a simple dislocation, the condyles are in contact; in a complex dislocation, the condyles are not in contact.

Urgent closed reduction and splinting are necessary for dislocations of the IP joints.

Follow-Up Evaluation

At the 1-week follow-up visit, the patient is encouraged to start with hand therapy (occupational therapy), to work on restoring normal motion and function.

REFERENCES

Bindra, R. R., & Foster, B. J. (2009). Management of proximal interphalangeal joint dislocations in athletes. *Hand Clinics, 25*(3), 423–435.

Leggit, J. C., & Meko, C. J. (2006). Acute finger injuries: Part II. Fractures, dislocations, and thumb injuries. *American Family Physician, 73*(5), 827–834.

Case Study 4.3: Acute Subungual Hematoma

Hardeep Singh and Craig M. Rodner

SETTING: URGENT CARE

Definition and Incidence

Subungual hematomas are an acute injury to the finger that occur as a result of crushing fingers between two objects. A collection of blood, or hematoma, develops between the nail and nail bed (Cohen, Schulze, & Nelson, 2007). Subungual hematomas can be associated with nail bed injury, DIP fracture, or dislocation.

Patient

An 18-year-old female presents to the emergency room after crushing her index finger while closing her car door. She reported immediate pain and swelling in her finger with discoloration of her nail. She denied any bleeding, numbness, or tingling. Her index finger motion is limited due to pain. She rates her pain as 7 out of 10 and any movement, or allowing the finger to be in a dependent position, increases the discomfort to 8 out of 10.

Social History

This female is a senior in high school. She is not an athlete, and lives at home with her two parents and two sisters. She works at a local coffee shop.

Physical Assessment

Physical examination reveals a pleasant female in no acute distress, but obvious discomfort. Inspection revealed swelling and erythema of her index finger, with a hematoma under the entirety of the nail bed. She was able to actively flex and extend both the PIP and DIP joints and was distally neurovascularly intact. There are no open lacerations.

Diagnostic Evaluations

Radiographs of her finger (anterior–posterior [AP], lateral, and oblique) did not reveal any fractures or dislocations.

Diagnosis

Subungual hematoma.

CLINICAL PEARL
Injuries with a hematoma involving less than 50% of the nail bed can be observed or drained by perforating the nail with a needle, depending upon the patient's discomfort level. Hematomas involving greater than 50% of the involved nail bed should be drained by removing the nail and inspecting for nail bed injuries.

Interventions

The patient received a digital nerve block with 1% lidocaine in the index finger. The nail was removed from the nail bed, the hematoma was evacuated, and a transverse laceration is noted on the nail bed. A nail bed repair is performed using absorbable stitches. The proximal nail fold is kept open using the patient's nail plate. She is placed in a dry sterile dressing and asked to follow up in clinic in 1 week.

CLINICAL PEARL
The degree of hematoma determines whether acute intervention to drain the hematoma is needed (Singer & Dagum, 2008).

Patient Education

Educate the patient to keep her dressing on until follow-up. Inquire about the patient's tetanus status, and provide a booster immunization as indicated. She is asked to rest her affected hand and keep it elevated to help with the swelling.

Follow-Up Evaluation

The patent returns for follow-up in 1 week. The dressing is removed and a radiograph is taken to assess healing. A light dressing is applied, and she is told to watch for signs of infection, including redness, drainage, or increasing pain. She follows up in 2 weeks and is discharged from care at that time.

REFERENCES

Cohen, P. R., Schulze, K. E., & Nelson, B. R. (2007). Subungual hematoma. *Dermatology Nursing, 19*(1), 83.

Singer, A. J., & Dagum, A. B. (2008). Current management of acute cutaneous wounds. *New England Journal of Medicine, 359*(10), 1037–1046.

Case Study 4.4: Chronic Trigger Finger

Hardeep Singh and Craig M. Rodner

SETTING: PRIMARY CARE

Definition and Incidence

Trigger fingers are a result of inflammation of flexor tendon sheath that leads to entrapment of the flexor tendon at the A-1 pulley (Adams & Habbu, 2015). This entrapment leads to symptomatic locking of the finger in a flexed position (Adams & Habbu, 2015). Risk factors for trigger fingers include diabetes mellitus, rheumatoid arthritis, and amyloidosis.

Patient

A 60-year-old diabetic female presents with the insidious onset of pain in the palm and painful clicking in her right ring finger for the past 3 to 4 months. She reported that it initially started with pain in the palm of her hand, progressing to clicking, and locking of her ring finger. She is able to unlock the finger; however, it interferes with her activities to daily living, and is becoming more bothersome.

Social History

She is a high school math teacher, married with adult children who do not live nearby. She is active with jazzercise and yoga.

Physical Assessment

On inspection, her physical examination reveals no obvious deformity, except for the position of her finger. With palpation, there is tenderness over the A-1 pulley as well as crepitus with ROM of her ring finger. The clicking and locking of her ring finger are reproduced upon exam, and a small nodule is palpable on the tendon sheath.

Diagnostic Evaluations

Radiographs are not indicated, as the diagnosis of trigger finger is a clinical diagnosis.

Diagnosis

Trigger finger, fourth finger.

Interventions

Conservative treatment options of splinting, nonsteroidal anti-inflammatory drugs (NSAIDs), steroid injections are discussed and the patient elects to have a trial of this treatment plan. A follow-up visit is scheduled at 4 weeks.

CLINICAL PEARLS

Trigger finger presents insidiously and is a result of stenosing tenosynovitis in the flexor tendon sheath (Saldana, 2001).

Initial symptoms include pain in the palm and tenderness at the A-1 pulley, which then progresses to catching of the digit. This is followed by progressive frequent locking of the digit, followed by the final stage of fixed locked digit.

Initial treatment can include splints, NSAIDs, and steroid injection into the tendon sheath. Definitive treatment involves release of the A-1 pulley.

Patient Education

Patient is asked to keep her postoperative dressing on until follow-up. She is asked to limit weight bearing on the affected hand. She is encouraged to move her fingers postoperatively.

Follow-Up Evaluation

When she returned at the fourth week, she stated that she did not receive much relief at all with the conservative measures that were tried. At this point, she decides to undergo a steroid injection of the ring finger. This injection is given with a corticosteroid (Kenalog or Depo-Medrol) at a dose of 1 mL along with 1 mL of lidocaine, right next to the area where she has a palpable nodule.

The patient experiences complete relief form the pain and triggering for several months. She undergoes repeat injections 4 and 8 months later, with diminishing relief from each subsequent injection. At this point, she is referred to the orthopedic surgeon and elects to undergo surgical release of the A-1 pulley. She is seen postoperatively and reported to be free of pain with no locking or clicking of her ring finger.

REFERENCES

Adams, J. E., & Habbu, R. (2015). Tendinopathies of the hand and wrist. *Journal of the American Academy of Orthopaedic Surgeons, 23*(12), 741–750.

Saldana, M. J. (2001). Trigger digits: Diagnosis and treatment. *Journal of the American Academy of Orthopaedic Surgeons, 9*(4), 246–252.

Case Study 4.5: Chronic Dupuytren's Contracture

Hardeep Singh and Craig M. Rodner

SETTING: PRIMARY CARE

Definition and Incidence

Dupuytren's contractures are an autosomal dominant condition with a high incidence in males in their 50s to 70s, of northern European descent (Blount & Felz, 2015).

Pathophysiology involves conversion of normal fascial bands into pathologic cords, which lead to contracture of the metacarpophalangeal (MCP), PIP, and DIP joints (Özkaya et al., 2010).

Patient

A 50-year-old male presents with painless fixed contracture of his right ring finger at the MCP joint. He reports it has been progressively getting worse over the past several months. He reports decreased ROM, with inability to fully extend his ring finger that interferes with his activities of daily living. He denies any trauma or injury that he can recall.

Social History

This 50-year-old gentleman is an accountant. He lives at home with his wife and a dog. He has two children who are married and live nearby.

Physical Assessment

Physical examination reveals contracture of his right ring MCP joint to 50 degrees without a PIP contracture. A cord is palpated in the palm of his hand. A Hueston's tabletop test is performed (ask patient to place palm flat on a table to assess MCP and PIP contracture) and the patient is unable to place his ring finger flat on the table. He is neurovascularly intact, with normal sensation throughout his hand and finger.

Diagnostic Evaluations

Clinical history and physical examination reveal that the patient is suffering from Dupuytren's contracture in his ring finger, leading to contracture of his MCP joint. Radiographs are not indicated to diagnose Dupuytren's disease.

Diagnosis

Dupuytren's contracture, ring finger, right hand.

Interventions

Nonoperative treatment options are discussed with the patient that include physical therapy to increase ROM and injection with collagenase into the cord to cause lysis and rupture of the cord. The patient elects for a collagenase injection to release the cord, and is referred to the hand specialist for this procedure. This is successful and full MCP extension is restored.

> ### CLINICAL PEARLS
>
> Dupuytren's contracture is a benign condition with development of fascial nodules and contractures in hand.
>
> Nodules and contractures lead to decreased ROM and can affect activities of daily living.

Patient Education

Instruct the patient that the recurrence rates are approximately 20% at 2 years, and that he should return if he has any further problems or recurrent symptoms.

REFERENCES

Blount, K., & Felz, M. (2015). Dupuytren disease: A hands-on disorder. *Clinical Advisor, 18*(7), 32–42.

Özkaya, O., Yesilada, A., Karsidag, S., Soydan, A., Ugurlu, K., & Bas, L. (2010). Dupuytren's contracture: Etiology, diagnosis and surgical treatment, retrospective analysis of ten years. *Turkiye Klinikleri Journal of Medical Sciences, 30*(2), 553–558.

Case Study 4.6: Chronic Osteoarthritis

Hardeep Singh and Craig M. Rodner

SETTING: PRIMARY CARE

Definition and Incidence

Osteoarthritis of the hands is prevalent in patients as they age (Altman & Gold, 2007). Signs of osteoarthritis include the following: joint space narrowing, osteophyte formation subchondral sclerosis, and subchondral cyst formation. There are a variety of causative mechanism of osteoarthritis, which include degenerative, traumatic, and inflammatory (Altman & Gold, 2007). Arthritis of interphalangeal (IP) joints is especially common as the DIP joints experience greater joint forces in the hand, therefore undergoing wear and tear.

Patient

The patient is a 70-year-old female who presents with pain and deformity in the PIP and DIP of her right index finger, and pain at the base of her thumb, and pain in the left third knuckle. She reports pain has been ongoing for several years; however, it has progressed to the point where she is unable to do her activities of daily living without pain. She has tried NSAIDs, and over-the-counter splint, which have now failed to provide her with relief.

Social History

She is a retired librarian who is widowed. She lives alone, and has two cats. She has a daughter and three grandchildren who live nearby.

Physical Examination

Physical examination of the right hand shows swelling of PIP (Bouchard's nodes) and DIP (Heberden's nodes) joints. ROM of PIP and DIP are limited due to pain. Examination of her thumb shows swelling at the carpometacarpal (CMC) joint; she has crepitus with ROM of the CMC joint. She has a painful CMC grind test (axial compression and circumduction of her thumb). On the left hand, she has pain with palpation over the third MCP joint.

Diagnostic Evaluations

Radiographs are taken of the left hand: AP, lateral, and oblique of hand (Figure 4.4), and demonstrate arthritis at the third MCP joint.

Radiographs are taken of the right thumb (Figure 4.5). The radiographs demonstrate joint space narrowing, osteophyte formation, and MCP joint hyperextension. And radiographs of the right hand (Figure 4.6) demonstrate arthritis of the second MCP joint.

Diagnosis

Osteoarthritis of the left hand, third MCP joint.
Osteoarthritis of the right hand, including the IP joint of the index finger and the CMC joint of the right thumb.

Interventions

All treatment options are discussed with the patient. A range of very conservative management with observation and NSAIDs (Naprosyn 500 mg with food twice a day) to surgical interventions is discussed. She decides to try the conservative measures and states that she will schedule a follow-up visit if symptoms persist.

Patient Education

Have a complete discussion with your patients regarding their ability to comfortably perform activities of daily living, and their need for intervention in order to be functional. Each patient's level of comfort and

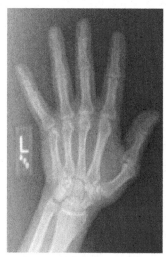

FIGURE 4.4 Radiograph of the posteroanterior (PA) of the left hand demonstrating third metacarpophalangeal arthritis.

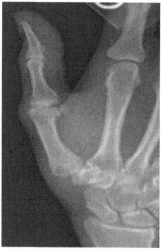

FIGURE 4.5 Radiograph of the posteroanterior (PA) of the right thumb demonstrating thumb carpometacarpal arthritis.

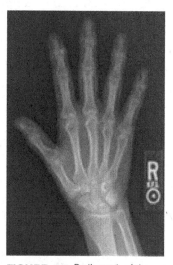

FIGURE 4.6 Radiograph of the posteroanterior (PA) of the right hand demonstrating severe second distal interphalangeal joint arthritis.

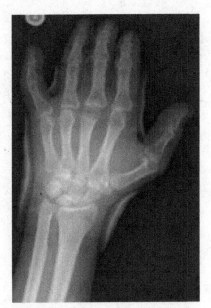

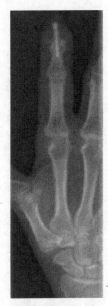

FIGURE 4.7 Radiograph of the postero-anterior (PA) of the left hand following third metacarpophalangeal arthroplasty.

FIGURE 4.8 Radiograph of the posteroanterior (PA) of the right hand demonstrating a second distal interphalangeal joint fusion.

ability to function should be considered in the treatment algorithm (Bukhave, la Cour, & Huniche, 2014).

Follow-Up Evaluation

Three months later, the patient called to follow up. She stated that the conservative measures were no longer allowing her to function, and she wanted to try something else.

She agreed to have a consultation with the hand surgeon, and elected to have surgical intervention. She underwent an arthroplasty of the third MCP (Figure 4.7). She returned 6 months later, and underwent a fusion of the right IP, which is indicated in patients who have debilitating pain (see Figure 4.8).

REFERENCES

Altman, R. D., & Gold, G. E. (2007). Atlas of individual radiographic features in osteoarthritis, revised. *Osteoarthritis and Cartilage, 15*, A1–A56.

Bukhave, E. B., la Cour, K., & Huniche, L. (2014). The meaning of activity and participation in everyday life when living with hand osteoarthritis. *Scandinavian Journal of Occupational Therapy, 21*(1), 24–30. doi:10.3109/11038128.2013.857428

SECTION II

Lower Extremity Cases

CHAPTER 5

Hip

Case Study 5.1: Acute Hip Dislocation

Karen M. Myrick

SETTING: URGENT CARE

Definition and Incidence

Anterior hip dislocations are infrequent, and caused by high-energy trauma, most often from a motor vehicle accident (Bastian, Turina, Siebenrock, & Keel, 2011). Recognition of the injury and expedient reduction are imperative for good patient outcomes.

Patient

Patient presents with his wife after being involved in a motor vehicle accident an hour prior to presenting. He is writhing in discomfort, and has to be helped into the center with the use of a wheel chair. His chief complaint is right hip pain, and he is unable to speak in full sentences.

Social History

This 28-year-old male is a construction worker with a large company near his hometown. He is married and does not have children.

Physical Assessment

The patient is a 28-year-old male who is in acute distress. He is 5'10" and weighs 220 lb, according to his wife. On inspection, his right leg is externally rotated and shortened. He has significant pain and is unable to communicate well. There are mild abrasions and small lacerations that are not actively bleeding on his knee of the right leg.

Diagnostic Evaluations

Radiographs are ordered in the room, and there is a dislocation of the right hip from the acetabulum.

Diagnosis

Anterior hip dislocation.

Interventions

The patient is given pain medication, morphine sulfate 10 mg, and a reduction is accomplished by placing him in a supine position, and using traction under the right knee in an upward and forward plane. After a clunk is felt, the patient is taken to x-ray for postreduction radiographs.

Patients who sustain hip dislocations should be evaluated with the consultation of an orthopedic surgeon. Many patients (65%–90%) will require arthroscopic evaluation and debridement for loose bodies within the joint (Keil, Vorburger, & Dahners, 2016).

Patient Education

Educate the patient on the importance of following up with orthopedics and limiting activity until such follow-up. Typically, the patient will be on crutches for a period of time, and begin touch-down weight bearing with the assistance of physical therapy. The potential long-term consequences of hip osteoarthritis, heterotopic ossification (HO), and avascular necrosis exist, and need to be discussed with patients and their families (Bastian et al., 2011).

Follow-Up Evaluation

Because this injury requires specialist consultation, the nurse practitioner may not follow up directly with the patient. If the nurse practitioner is in a setting where nurses work collaboratively with an orthopedic surgeon, the nurse may have the opportunity to directly follow up and even perform the preoperative and postoperative care of the patient, and may even be in a position to assist in the operating room. For the primary care nurse practitioner, it is likely the patient would return after the specialist consultation and any surgical intervention and rehabilitation has been completed, as the patient has been discharged from the specialist's care. It is also highly likely that the nurse practitioner will care for patients on occasion who have sustained a hip dislocation at some point in their history. Being astute to the potential sequelae is important for early recognition and treatment.

REFERENCES

Bastian, J. D., Turina, M., Siebenrock, K. A., & Keel, M. B. (2011). Long-term outcome after traumatic anterior dislocation of the hip. *Archives of Orthopaedic & Trauma Surgery*, *131*(9), 1273–1278.

Keil, L. G., Vorburger, M. S., & Dahners, L. E. (2016). Junk in the joint: A trend for arthroscopic debridement to improve outcomes following closed reduction of traumatic hip dislocation. *Trauma*, *18*(1), 35–39. doi:10.1177/1460408615606754

Case Study 5.2: Acute Hip Labral Tear

Karen M. Myrick

SETTING: URGENT CARE

Definition and Incidence

The acetabular labrum is a structure within the hip joint that is fibrous cartilage, and attaches to the edge of the acetabulum (Tian, Wang, Zheng, & Ren, 2014). The prevalence of labral tears in painful hips of young athletic individuals is reported as 22% to 55% (Skendzel & Philippon, 2013).

Patient

Patient presents with the chief complaint of left hip pain. She describes an insidious onset of hip and groin pain that is worse with certain dance moves that she performs, including twisting while weight bearing on this left leg. The pain is a 2 out of 10, 10 being the worst, at rest, and she experiences occasional episodes of catching, which she defines as an 8 out of 10. She has just completed a busy season while performing, and describes the pain as intolerable when it occurs, and becoming more frequent. There is no associated swelling or numbness, but she describes her leg as feeling weak and achy after an episode of catching. Pain is occasionally associated with a limp, favoring the left leg. She tried ibuprofen, 600 mg two times a day over the past 2 weeks, but really did not find this to make a difference in the discomfort.

Social History

This 11-year-old ballerina has been dancing for the past 6 years at a very high level. She lives at home with her mother and two siblings, a brother and sister. She is in the fifth grade.

CLINICAL PEARL

Labral tears are associated with painful catching episodes, whereas a snapping hip is typically noisy and felt by the patient; however, they are not painful (Zini, Munegato, De Benedetto, Carraro, & Bigoni, 2013).

Physical Assessment

The patient is an 11-year-old female who is in no acute distress; she is ambulatory without an antalgic gait. She is 5'0" and weighs 102 lb. On inspection, there is no gross deformity noted. With palpation, she has no bony tenderness, and no palpable snapping or clunking with range of motion (ROM). ROM is full with flexion to 125 degrees, extension at 30 degrees, abduction at 45 degrees, and adduction at 20 degrees. She has external rotation to 45 degrees and internal rotation to 35 degrees, but internal rotation is painful. With The Hip Internal Rotation with Distraction (THIRD) testing she has relief of her symptoms, and therefore a positive THIRD test (Myrick & Nissen, 2013). Hip abductors, adductors, quadriceps, and hamstring strength are 5 out of 5.

Diagnostic Evaluations

A radiograph was not obtained, due to the lack of yield on information that would be likely in this patient. Magnetic resonance imagery with arthrogram (MRA) was obtained. The MRA demonstrated a hip labral tear.

CLINICAL PEARL
An MRA may not be necessary, depending on the unique patient presentation. The positive predictive value of the THIRD test is 100% (Myrick & Feinn, 2014).

Diagnosis

Hip labral tear.

Interventions

The patient was referred to an orthopedic surgeon for evaluation and consultation. The suggestion was for arthroscopic debridement of the labral tear, followed by physical therapy.

Patient Education

It is very important to educate both the patient and her parents about the likelihood of the diagnosis of labral tear given her history and physical examination findings. The information obtained with an MRA is likely to assist with surgical intervention, including the evaluation for underlying bony abnormalities that might need to be addressed surgically.

Follow-Up Evaluation

Because this injury requires surgical consultation, the nurse practitioner may not follow up directly with the patient. If the nurse practitioner is in a setting where nurses work collaboratively with an orthopedic surgeon, the nurse may perform the preoperative and postoperative care of the patient, and may even be in a position to assist in the operating room. For the primary care nurse practitioner, it is likely the patient would return after the surgical intervention and rehabilitation has been completed, and the patient has been discharged from the specialist's care

REFERENCES

Myrick, K. M., & Feinn, R. (2014). Internal and external validity of THIRD test for hip labral tears . . . hip internal rotation with distraction. *Journal for Nurse Practitioners, 10*(8), 540–544. doi:10.1016/j.nurpra.2014.06.021

Myrick, K. M., & Nissen, C. W. (2013). THIRD test: Diagnosing hip labral tears with a new physical examination technique . . . the hip internal rotation with distraction (THIRD). *Journal for Nurse Practitioners, 9*(8), 501–505. doi:10.1016/j.nurpra.2013.06.008

Skendzel, J. G., & Philippon, M. J. (2013). Management of labral tears of the hip in young patients. *Orthopedic Clinics of North America, 44*(4), 477–487. doi:10.1016/j.ocl.2013.06.003

Tian, C., Wang, J., Zheng, Z., & Ren, A. (2014). 3.0T conventional hip MR and hip MR arthrography for the acetabular labral tears confirmed by arthroscopy. *European Journal of Radiology, 83*(10), 1822–1827. doi:10.1016/j.ejrad.2014.05.034

Zini, R., Munegato, D., De Benedetto, M., Carraro, A., & Bigoni, M. (2013). Endoscopic iliotibial band release in snapping hip. *Hip International, 23*(2), 225–232. doi:10.5301/HIP.2013.10878

Case Study 5.3: Acute Greater Trochanteric Bursitis

Susan H. Lynch

SETTING: PRIMARY CARE

Definition and Incidence

Greater trochanteric bursitis or greater trochanteric hip pain describes lateral hip that is insidious in onset and chronic in nature. Muscles and tendons that attach to the greater trochanter and bursae which serve to protect the soft tissue are located in this region. The term "bursitis" in the diagnosis implies inflammation in the bursa; however, this is often not found (Mallow & Nazarian, 2014). Complaints of hip pain have an incidence of 10% to 25%, are more common in those older than 60, and more prevalent in women than men (Mulligan, 2015).

Patient

Patient presents with right hip pain which has been present for approximately 1 year. He complains that the pain is intermittent and denies any associated trauma with its onset. He does admit to playing golf and carrying his golf bag as he walks. He denies any pain while walking and carrying his bag but states that the pain occurs primarily at night. It wakes him from his sleep and prevents him from sleeping on the right side or his back. He denies radiation to the back, thigh, knee, or calf. He denies walking with a limp or any associated leg weakness or foot drop. He denies pain at rest and when the pain does occur it usually is 5 out of 10, reported as an ache. He does report some relief with nonsteroidal anti-inflammatory drugs (NSAIDs) but states that the pain returns. The patient was treated conservatively and encouraged to continue with NSAIDs as necessary to relieve pain, and to ice after activity. After 8 to 12 weeks the patient returned to the provider without resolution of his symptoms.

Social History

The patient is a 59-year-old male who is employed in an office setting. He is active and exercises regularly including weight-bearing exercises several times a week. He plays golf and carries his golf bag three times a week during the spring, summer, and fall. He lives at home with his wife.

Physical Assessment

On examination, the patient is a well-appearing 59-year-old male in no apparent distress. He is alert and oriented to time, place, and date. He ambulates with a steady, symmetric gait. On examination, no deformities are noted. Skin is warm and intact without edema or erythema. Hips are symmetric. Slight pain to palpation over the greater trochanter was elicited with no pain over surrounding soft tissue. There is no snapping, popping, clicking, or groin pain with ROM. He has full ROM to flexion/extension, abduction/adduction both active and passive. He has 5 out of 5 leg strength bilaterally, full sensation to sharp/dull, 2+ pulses throughout.

Diagnostic Evaluations

Due to the patient's complaint of persistent yet not progressive symptoms, the patient was referred for x-ray. The results showed no acute trauma or fracture, no irregularities of the greater trochanter, but essentially normal hip joint with slight degenerative changes consistent with age.

Diagnosis

Greater trochanteric bursitis.

Interventions

With negative radiographic results and the patient's continued complaint of symptoms with conservative treatment of ice, rest, and NSAIDs, the patient was referred to orthopedic surgery. The orthopedic surgeon did not order additional imaging but continued NSAIDs and physical therapy for 6 weeks.

In some cases, it is reasonable and appropriate for the patient to receive steroid injection into the joint (Mulligan, 2015). Less common is surgical intervention, which is used for those cases that do not respond to conservative treatment, physical therapy, or corticosteroid injections into the bursa (Mallow & Nazarian, 2014).

Patient Education

Educate your patients to be fully informed of all options for intervention and therapy. They should also be fully informed of prognosis. The patient should be a participant in the decision making of additional treatments with the goal of treatment being to return the patient to maximum functionality for the diagnosis.

Follow-Up Evaluation

The patient reports at his last annual exam that he has continued with exercises as prescribed by physical therapy and at this time remains pain free. He continues to be pain free and takes part in the activities he enjoys.

REFERENCES

Mallow, M., & Nazarian, L. (2014). Greater trochanteric pain syndrome and treatment. *Physics Medicine and Rehabilitation Clinics of North America, 25,* 279–289. doi:10.1016/j.pmr.2014.01.009

Mulligan, E., Middleton, E., & Brunette, M. (2015). Evaluation and management of greater trochanter pain syndrome. *Physical Therapy in Sport, 16,* 205–214. doi:10.1016/j/ptsp.2014.11.002

Case Study 5.4: Chronic Osteoarthritis

Susan D'Agostino

SETTING: PRIMARY CARE

Definition and Incidence

Osteoarthritis (OA) is defined as a "joint failure" or degeneration due to pathologic changes over time. Hip arthritis is a common problem in the older patient population.

Patient

Patient presents with the chief complaint of "left hip pain" off and on for 7 months. He complains of pain in the left groin, around the left hip, and buttock. Intermittently, the pain radiates down the left thigh to the knee. He denies any acute trauma and admits to decreasing his running and cycling distance secondary to pain. He describes the pain in the left hip is better upon awakening in the morning but worsens as the day progresses. He is experiencing daily pain, with the worst being 6 out of 10 on the pain scale. He was initially seen by his primary care provider and treated conservatively with a pharmacologic agent Naprosyn (nonsteroidal anti-inflammatory) at a dose of 500 mg twice a day. After 6 weeks, the patient was reevaluated. This exam revealed no pain relief was attained with the prescribed medication and the patient reported a decrease in strength of the left leg. He reports no limping but increased stiffness after long periods of sitting to standing position. Within the past few days, he reports some difficulty putting his shoes and socks on.

Social History

These symptoms prompted the primary care provider to refer the patient for x-rays of the left hip and to physical therapy. The patient is very concerned with his prognosis. He has a strong desire to return to his regular activities. Currently, he is working full time.

Physical Assessment

On physical examination, the patient is a 63-year-old male with no past medical history, who is alert and oriented to person, place, and time and noticeably in pain. He walks with a stable symmetric gait. On the exam table, both hips and the surrounding skin were assessed and noted to be warm and of equal temperature bilaterally. No tenderness was noted when palpating both the left and left greater trochanter. There is limited ROM and pain with lateral rotation of the left hip. There is less left hip discomfort with flexion and external rotation. The assessment of the patient's distal neuro-vascular status is intact bilaterally.

Diagnostic Evaluation

Radiographs were obtained of the anterior–posterior (AP) and frog lateral views of the hips (Figures 5.1–5.3). Progression of arthritis of his left hip was shown.

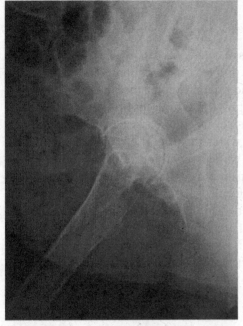

FIGURE 5.1 Frog lateral radiograph of the left hip demonstrating degenerative joint disease.

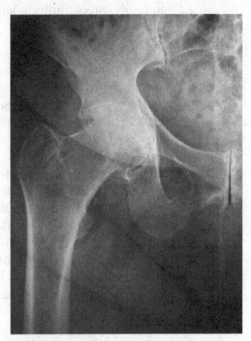

FIGURE 5.2 Anterior–posterior radiograph of the left hip demonstrating degenerative joint disease.

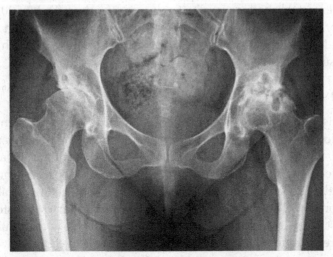

FIGURE 5.3 Anterior–posterior view of both (bilateral) hips.

No acute fracture or dislocation is identified. The patient's left hip appears to have bone-on-bone superolateral arthritis with peripheral osteophytes and calcification of the labrum and capsule, which can be demonstrated in Figure 5.1. This may even represent a calcifying loose chondral fragment. Incidentally, his left hip appears to have 50% loss of the cartilage joint space.

Diagnosis

Progressive (chronic) osteoarthritis (degenerative joint disease) of left hip and early osteoarthritis in left hip.

Interventions

Once you have made the diagnosis of progressive (chronic) osteoarthritis of the hip, there are several treatment options for the patient to consider. In the setting of primary care, physical and pharmacologic therapies were initiated but due to the patient's increased physical symptoms and poor response to prescribed Naprosyn, you can consider use of an assistance walking device (cane) as needed and physical or water therapy. The patient feels he "has been down this route before and wants something done." Another medical intervention presented to this patient is cortisone injections to decrease inflammation. The patient was informed about potential side effects that may occur with intraarticular corticosteroid injection procedure such as: pain with injection, postinjection flare, skin pigment changes, fat atrophy, and joint infection (Kruse, 2008). The patient decided upon an intraarticular corticosteroid injection into the left hip which was scheduled and was performed with fluoroscopic guidance.

Patient Education

For your patient to make an informed decision about treatment options, he or she should understand that once chronic osteoarthritis in the hip has been established, generally it worsens over time (Dubin, 2016). The goal of any treatment option is for the patient to be relieved of pain and to decrease their disability. Once achieved, the effort to improve strength and function to resume their desired activities of daily living is the goal.

Follow-Up Evaluation

This patient achieved pain-free status within hours of the injection. He was told to follow up as needed if or when the left hip causes pain or disability. Short-term reduction of pain is the goal of intraarticular corticosteroid injections. Some patients may experience less pain within hours, while with others the pain may return after the preprocedure local anesthetic has worn off. The duration of time the intraarticular corticosteroid injections last varies from patient to patient. It may last weeks to months. Most health care providers limit the amount of cortisone injections given in a specific joint to decrease the potential of further injury within the joint (Cole & Schumacher, 2005; Masala, 2010).

The patient was free of left hip pain and disability for 13 months. He followed up with the orthopedist for consultation, and for a possible second intraarticular corticosteroid injection. Repeat x-rays revealed increased loss of articular cartilage to the left hip. At this time, the patient was informed to consider a future left hip replacement.

REFERENCES

Cole, B. J., & Schumacher, R. H. (2005). Injectable corticosteroids in modern practice. *Journal of the American Academy of Orthopaedic Surgeons, 13*(1), 37–46.

Dubin, A. (2016). Managing osteoarthritis and other chronic musculoskeletal pain disorders. *Medical Clinics of North America, 100*, 143–150.

Kruse, D. W. (2008). Intraarticular cortisone injection for osteoarthritis of the hip. Is it effective? Is it safe? *Current Reviews in Musculoskeletal Medicine, 1*(3–4), 227–233.

Masala, S., Fiori, R., Bartolucci, D. A., Mammucari, M., Angelopoulos, G., Massari, F., & Simonetti, G. (2010). Diagnostic and therapeutic joint injections. *Seminars in Interventional Radiology, 27*(2), 160–171.

Case Study 5.5: Groin Muscle Strain

Scott A. Myrick and Karen M. Myrick

SETTING: URGENT CARE OR PRIMARY CARE

Definition and Incidence

One of the more common injuries that athletes and nonathletes alike can experience is that of groin muscle strain (Maffey & Emery, 2007). A groin strain is described as a pull or strain of the adductor muscles of the hip (Chang, Turcotte, & Pearsall, 2009).

Patient

In the office is a 17-year-old male hockey player from a local high school. He complains of an inner thigh pain sharp in nature that began when he was skating 2 days ago. As the patient has practice each afternoon after school, he reported to the ice early to skate around. He was playing with a teammate and went to change directions abruptly when he felt a sharp pain in his leg. Even though the pain was sharp, he continued to try to skate and even make it through his entire 2-hour practice. To no avail, he had to sit as he was unable to skate with any speed.

The patient mentions he thought he'd be better the next day but it was worse, stiff and sorer with limited motion in his hip. Worried, he figured he needed medical attention.

Social History

This 17-year-old presents with his father, and is obviously frustrated in his inability to play hockey, but he is a charming young man with a good attitude. He is a very active student who has a very good academic record. After graduating high school, he plans to attend college and continue to play hockey on scholarship. A very dedicated athlete, he mentions his exercise routine typically includes 3 to 4 days a week, even in season. He does not drink or smoke, has no siblings, and lives at home with both parents.

> ### CLINICAL PEARL
>
> With many muscle strains, flexibility, overtraining, and training imbalances can all contribute to injury.

Physical Assessment

He is 5'8", 170 lb. He is in some distress but mentions it hurts only when he moves his affected leg. Walking is generally okay, but anything faster such as jogging, running, or skating are out of the question. He did present with a slight limp, however. With inspection, there is some bruising that begins high up the inner thigh and tracks down toward the medial knee stopping about 6"short. Upon palpation, there is pain elicited along the medial thigh from the mid muscle belly proximally to the right pubis symphasis, ending just prior.

ROM shows a very inflexible athlete generally. He has equal and bilateral normal hip internal and external rotation but with a passive straight leg raise in a supine position, he has 65 degrees with some effort. Lying prone, his heel cannot touch his buttocks, and he demonstrates 100 degrees of knee flexion. He has a negative Scour test but a positive Thomas test performed supine indicating tight hip flexors also.

Strength testing demonstrates 5 out of 5 hip flexion, hip extension, hip abduction, and knee extension, all without pain. Knee flexion is strong but does elicit some pain at the inner thigh. Hip adduction elicits the greatest pain and is weak, 3 out of 5.

Diagnostic Evaluations

A radiograph was obtained to look for the presence of any fracture avulsion near the pubis symphasis. There is no visible evidence of any fracture.

Diagnosis

Right groin strain.

Interventions

Despite pleadings from the athlete, it is strongly advised he abstain from practice, games, and any physical training that involves the affected area for 4 to 6 weeks. During this time, rest is important to allow muscle fibers to heal. Once a pain-free resisted hip adduction test can be performed, gentle stretching, and moderate exercise for the lower extremity such as stationary cycling can be initiated. To assist with his recovery, he is instructed on the use of ice for pain. He may use NSAIDs if needed which may also help with healing.

For this treatment protocol, a regimen of strict physical therapy is prescribed to allow the patient to adhere to the restrictions. Follow-up with the provider at the end of the 4- to 6-week time frame is recommended to gauge progress.

Patient Education

It is particularly important with muscle strains that the patient understand no aggravating activity should be performed. This can serve only to lengthen the amount of time needed for recovery. It can also increase the amount of scarring present at the injury site making it more likely a recurrent injury may show itself later on.

Educate the patient that a proper warm-up, cool down, and stretching routine is essential. It's advised the athlete spend at least 15 to 20 minutes warming up before each practice and game and the same after each practice and game. During this time, a vigorous stretching routine is prescribed that will help prevent muscle strains. Given the extreme lack of flexibility, it's suggested this routine be performed daily, regardless of play and practice schedule. Provide your patient with a note stating this information, which is also for the benefit of the coach.

Follow-Up Evaluation

Once the patient has completed the treatment regimen and is pain free, he was reevaluated to ensure he could perform the necessary tasks to play hockey. He was able to do so, and allowed a graduated return to competition.

REFERENCES

Chang, R., Turcotte, R., & Pearsall, D. (2009). Hip adductor muscle function in forward skating. *Sports Biomechanics, 8*(3), 212–222.

Maffey, L., & Emery, C. (2007). What are the risk factors for groin strain injury in sport? *Sports Medicine, 37*(10), 881–894.

Case Study 5.6: Chronic Heterotopic Ossification

Karen M. Myrick

SETTING: PRIMARY CARE

Definition and Incidence

Heterotopic ossification (HO) is typically found in areas around a joint following trauma, and is the benign formation of new bone in the soft tissues or external surface of an affected bone (Adams, 2014). Approximately 75% of cases are the result of trauma (Adams, 2014).

Patient

Patient presents with the chief complaint of left hip pain. He describes an insidious onset of hip and groin pain that is worse with exercise and has been present for the past 5 or more years. The pain is a 0 out of 10 at rest, and he experiences occasional episodes of significant pain, most recently while taking kickboxing classes and performing kicks. This discomfort is described as pinching, which he defines as an 8 out of 10. The discomfort is causing him to alter the way that he kicks in his martial arts, and becoming more frequent. There is no associated swelling, numbness, weakness, and no locking or catching. He describes the hip as feeling achy after an episode of pinching discomfort. Pain is not associated with a limp, and he has tried yoga and stretching to alleviate the discomfort, which help minimally.

Social History

This 38-year-old man is self-employed as a financial advisor. He lives at home with his wife and 6-year-old daughter.

CLINICAL PEARL

When a patient presents with atraumatic reduced hip function and groin pain during exercise, the nurse practitioner should consider HO as a differential diagnosis (Berry, Majeed, Deall, Arumugam, & Remedios, 2015).

Physical Assessment

The patient is a 38-year-old male who is in no acute distress; he is ambulatory without an antalgic gait. He is 6'1" and weighs 202 lb. On inspection, there is no gross deformity noted. With palpation, he has no bony tenderness, and no palpable snapping or clunking with ROM. ROM demonstrates full flexion to 125 degrees, but a pinch is felt at the extreme of motion. Extension is full at 30 degrees, abduction at 45 degrees, and adduction at 20 degrees. He has external rotation to 45 degrees and internal rotation is significantly limited to 5 degrees, and not painful. Internal rotation is met with a significantly solid end point. Hip abductors, adductors, quadriceps, and hamstring strength are 5 out of 5.

Diagnostic Evaluations

A radiograph was obtained, and revealed HO in the left hip.

Diagnosis

HO in the left hip.

Interventions

Treatment options were discussed with the patient, and included activity modification, and referral to an orthopedic surgeon for evaluation and consultation. The suggestion was for surgical debridement of the HO, followed by physical therapy.

Patient Education

Educate the patient on all treatment options from conservative management to surgical intervention. In this case, the treatment will be guided by the patient's perceived quality of life and the effect the condition has on his or her activities of daily living.

Follow-Up Evaluation

This patient was followed up 7 months later on his routine physical examination. At this time, he was 5 months out from the surgical intervention to remove the HO and he had completed a 6-week course of physical therapy. He reported following a home exercise program, and returning to his workouts, including the martial arts, without pain.

REFERENCES

Adams, L. (2014). Heterotopic ossification. *Radiation Therapist, 23*(1), 27–48.

Berry, B., Majeed, H., Deall, C., Arumugam, G., & Remedios, I. D. (2015). Large ossification mass causing groin pain and limited hip function. *Trauma, 17*(3), 235–237. doi:10.1177/1460408614562495

CHAPTER 6

Knee

Case Study 6.1: Acute Anterior Cruciate Ligament Tear

Karen M. Myrick

SETTING: ORTHOPEDIC URGENT CARE

Definition and Incidence

The anterior cruciate ligament (ACL) is one of the most common traumatic knee injuries. The ACL is one of the primary stabilizers in the knee, and prevents anterior displacement of the tibia on the femur. An estimated 120,000 ACL injuries affect athletes in the United States alone annually (Beynnon et al., 2014).

Patient

Patient presents with the chief complaint of left "knee pain." He describes a history of playing football at his high school 2 days ago. He states, "I was running down field when the whistle blew; I stopped as the play ended, and was going to go back to the huddle. No one was right near me; suddenly, I felt a pop, and it felt as if my knee went around in a circle. I fell to the ground." He was helped off the field by the athletic trainer, coach, and team doctor, but walked under his own power. He describes the swelling as immediate, and this has slightly receded over the past 2 days. Discomfort is well located in the left knee and mild, rated as a 2 out of 10. Pain is associated with a limp, favoring the left leg. He has been using a short, hinged brace that was placed by the athletic trainer, and this helps him to feel a little more stable. He tried ibuprofen, 800 mg once or twice, but really did not find this to make a difference in the swelling or discomfort. Applying ice 20 minutes four to five times a day has been beneficial in reducing both swelling and discomfort.

Social History

This 17-year-old male is in his senior year of high school, and this was his first game of the season. He has been recruited to play at the collegiate level. His anger, frustration, and situational depression are evident throughout the visit. It is likely that given the injury, he, along with his parents, will need to determine the course of treatment, which can be nonoperative or operative. If he chooses operative treatment, the rehabilitation will include approximately 6 months of physical therapy prior to allowing him a return to play status.

CLINICAL PEARL

The majority of ACL tears occur from a noncontact mechanism of injury (Waldén et al., 2015).

Physical Assessment

The patient is a 17-year-old male who is in no acute distress, but demonstrates hesitancy and some discomfort throughout the physical examination. He is 6'0" and weighs 213 lb. His gait is antalgic, demonstrating a shortened stance phase on the left knee, and weight bearing with approximately 15 degrees of flexion. On inspection, there is a moderate joint effusion, and no open cuts or abrasions. With palpation, the moderate joint effusion is confirmed with a positive buldge sign and fullness noted in the suprapatellar pouch. Range of motion in the knee is from 5 to 130, and he prefers to hold his knee at a slightly flexed position of approximately 10 degrees. There is no solid block with motion, but a description of "tightness" and "stiffness" from the patient with extremes of motion. A positive Lachman's test is elicited, with increased translation and a soft end point on this left knee. There is also a positive flexion pinch test, which correlates with tenderness to palpation of the medial posterior joint line. With valgus stressing, there is increased anterior translation of the tibia at 30 degrees, but not at 0 degrees; varus stressing is solid, without increased motion. Anterior drawer is positive, and a Pivot shift test is equivocal; no clunk is elicited at 20 to 30 degrees of flexion with a valgus force and the foot in internal rotation. Quadriceps and hamstring strength are 4 out of 5 and seemingly inhibited by discomfort. There are no focal neurological deficits in the left lower extremity.

Diagnostic Evaluations

A radiograph was not obtained, due to the lack of yield on information that would be likely in this patient. An MRI was obtained. The MRI demonstrated a completely torn ACL, and a medial meniscus tear (see Figure 6.1).

Diagnosis

ACL tear and medial meniscus tear.

Interventions

The patient was placed into a long leg, hinged knee brace, locked at 20 degrees of flexion, and he was given crutches to use until his follow-up with the orthopedic surgeon. Follow-up within 3 to 5 days was arranged with the surgeon for discussion of all options, including surgical intervention. A copy of the patient's MRI was given to him to bring to the consultation.

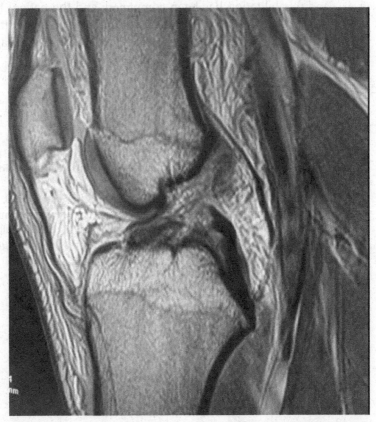

FIGURE 6.1 An MRI demonstrating an anterior cruciate ligament tear and medial meniscus tear.

Patient Education

It is very important to educate both the patient and his parents about the possible treatment options for treatment of ACL tears, which include operative and nonoperative management. Equally important is educating the patient and his family to avoid activity, especially cutting and pivoting maneuvers, until they follow up with the orthopedic surgeon. The potential for further damage to the knee joint is high, including damage to the articular cartilage with the shearing forces that will be present without an intact ACL.

Follow-Up Evaluation

As this injury requires surgical consultation, it is possible that the nurse practitioner may not follow up directly with the patient. If the nurse practitioner is in a setting working collaboratively with an orthopedic surgeon, the nurse may perform the preoperative and postoperative care of the patient, and may be in a position to assist in the operating room. For the primary care nurse practitioner, it is likely the patient will return after surgical intervention and rehabilitation has been completed, and the patient is discharged from the specialist. Also highly likely is that the nurse practitioner will care for patients in a variety of stages of ACL injury and rehabilitation.

REFERENCES

Beynnon, B. D., Vacek, P. M., Newell, M. K., Tourville, T. W., Smith, H. C., Shultz, S. J., & Johnson, R. J. (2014). The effects of level of competition, sport, and sex on the incidence of first-time noncontact anterior cruciate ligament injury. *American Journal of Sports Medicine, 42*(8), 1806–1812.

Waldén, M., Krosshaug, T., Bjørneboe, J., Einar Andersen, T., Faul, O., Hägglund, M., & Andersen, T. E. (2015). Three distinct mechanisms predominate in non-contact anterior cruciate ligament injuries in male professional football players: A systematic video analysis of 39 cases. *British Journal of Sports Medicine, 49*(22), 1–10.

Case Study 6.2: Acute Meniscus Tear

Karen M. Myrick

SETTING: ORTHOPEDIC URGENT CARE

Definition and Incidence

The meniscus is the C-shaped shock-absorbing cartilage in the tibio-femoral joint of the knee. Meniscal tears are the most common knee injury, and seen across the life span (Xu & Zhao, 2015).

Patient

Patient presents with the chief complaint of right "knee pain." She describes a history of playing with her 6-year-old daughter 5 days ago, kicking a soccer ball around in the backyard. When she attempted to kick the ball with her left foot toward the goal, her planted and slightly bent right leg twisted and she felt discomfort. She thinks that she may have heard or felt a "pop." She did not fall, but was unable to continue playing. She walked home with her daughter, and iced her knee. The ice helped the discomfort that was 5 out of 10, 10 being the worst. There was no swelling that night, any bruising, or ecchymosis. When she woke up the following day, she noticed that there was a moderate amount of swelling in the knee, which has decreased slightly, but is still present. Discomfort is located in the right knee, medial side, and mild, rated as 2 out of 10. She has been taking Naprosyn 500 mg twice a day since, which helps the aching discomfort, but has not resolved the swelling.

CLINICAL PEARL

The patient with a meniscus tear usually will not have swelling immediately following the injury. It is most common for any swelling related to a meniscus tear to develop within 48 hours. This is in contrast to the ACL tear, where an immediate joint effusion (hemarthrosis) is commonplace. Note that both problems may present with the patient feeling a "pop" during the time of injury.

Social History

This 39-year-old female is a first-grade teacher and mother of two. She is married and has a supportive husband who works as an accountant. She is active and was training for a marathon in 4 months.

> ### CLINICAL PEARL
>
> Meniscus tears can occur in a vascular or an avascular portion of the meniscus. When the tear is in the area of the meniscus that is avascular, it is likely part of the constellation of symptoms that are associated with degenerative joint disease. When the tear is in the vascular (red) zone, the tear should be repaired as soon as possible, due to the likelihood for healing if treated urgently (Sancheti, Razi, Ramanathan, & Yung, 2010). An MRI can assist in determining the area of the meniscus tear.

Physical Assessment

The patient is a 39-year-old female who is not in any acute distress, but has some tenderness with examination. She is 5'5" and weighs 131 lb. Her gait demonstrates a normal swing and stance phase, and is not antalgic. On inspection, there is a mild joint effusion, and no open cuts or abrasions. Palpation reveals a mild joint effusion with a positive bulge sign and slight fullness noted in the suprapatellar pouch, and point tenderness to palpation of the medial posterior joint line. Range of motion in the knee is full from 0 to 135 degrees. A positive flexion pinch test is identified, with the patient feeling pain over the medial aspect of the knee with full flexion. There is no ligamentous laxity with varus or valgus stressing, and a negative Lachman's test and negative Anterior drawer test. Quadriceps and hamstring strengths are 5 out of 5 and equal to the noninjured leg. There are no focal neurological deficits in the left lower extremity.

Diagnostic Evaluations

A radiograph of the right knee was obtained, evaluating the anteroposterior (AP) view, the lateral view, and a sunrise view. Radiographs demonstrate mild degenerative joint disease with medial joint space narrowing, a small osteophyte on the medial femoral condyle, and no fracture or dislocation, as shown in Figure 6.2.

Diagnosis

Medial meniscus tear.

Interventions

The patient was discharged with a hinged knee brace for support and comfort.

Patient Education

Education for patients with a meniscus tear will assist them in having a better understanding of their injury and their treatment options. The potential

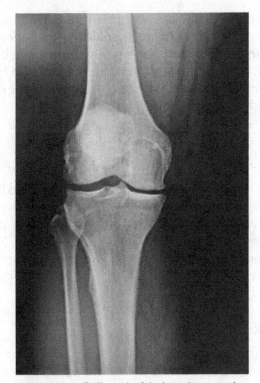

FIGURE 6.2 Radiograph of the knee demonstrating mild degenerative changes.

for further damage to the knee joint is present, and limiting high impact or cutting and pivoting activities in the acute phase is recommended until follow-up.

Follow-Up Evaluation

Follow-up is recommended at 2 weeks, to assess the patient's symptoms and level of impact these symptoms are having on activities of daily living. At the 2-week mark, this patient continued to have mechanical symptoms, those of locking, catching, and giving way. Her effusion had subsided. Because of her symptomatology, an MRI was obtained. The MRI demonstrated a small tear of the medial meniscus. Treatment options at this time were presented to the patient. She could undergo a trial of formalized physical therapy to strengthen the muscles surrounding the knee and the hip and core; she could try an injection with hyaluronic acid (Synvisc, Hyalgan, Gel-One); or she could opt for a consultation with an orthopedic surgeon for possible arthroscopic debridement. She opted for a 6-week course of physical therapy, and a return visit for follow-up.

For the primary care nurse practitioner, he or she will order and assess the effectiveness of physical therapy, having the patient return at the end of a 6-week course. It is also likely that the primary care nurse practitioner will learn the techniques of intra-articular injection, and perform this in his or her office. The treatment is guided by the patient's symptoms and tolerance of those symptoms. The nurse practitioner will care for patients who have had meniscus injuries, and a keen knowledge of the options and treatment plans is important. This patient returned at the 6-week postphysical therapy mark and had no further discomfort.

CLINICAL PEARL

It is important for the nurse practitioner to educate the patient about all of his or her treatment options. The effectiveness of surgical intervention is debated, and any surgery does carry risk (Kamimura, Umehara, Takahashi, Aizawa, & Itoi, 2015). Therefore, a treatment algorithm that includes noninvasive options should be employed, and carried out in a step-wise fashion.

REFERENCES

Kamimura, M., Umehara, J., Takahashi, A., Aizawa, T., & Itoi, E. (2015). Medial meniscus tears morphology and related clinical symptoms in patients with medial knee osteoarthritis. *Knee Surgery, Sports Traumatology, Arthroscopy, 23*(1), 158–163.

Sancheti, P., Razi, M., Ramanathan, E. S., & Yung, P. (2010). Injuries around the knee—Symposium. *British Journal of Sports Medicine, 44*(S1), i1.

Xu, C., & Zhao, J. (2015). A meta-analysis comparing meniscal repair with meniscectomy in the treatment of meniscal tears: The more meniscus, the better outcome? *Knee Surgery, Sports Traumatology, Arthroscopy, 23*(1), 164–170.

Case Study 6.3: Acute Patellar Dislocation

Karen M. Myrick

SETTING: ORTHOPEDIC URGENT CARE

Definition and Incidence

The patella of the knee can disarticulate, or dislocate, and this usually occurs laterally. The injury is more common in active children and young adults, with the incidence decreasing with age (Koh & Stewart, 2014). Patellar dislocations account for approximately 3% of all knee injuries and the incidence is one in 1,000 (Koh & Stewart, 2014).

Patient

Patient presents with the chief complaint of severe left "knee pain" and deformity. He describes a history of hiking with his family at a nearby state park. He was descending a steeply graded hill when he slipped on leaves. He notes that his knee cap went out of place and he fell to the ground screaming in pain. He was able to make it out of the woods and to the car, but had to be helped by two other hikers. He states that the pain is sharp in quality and it is difficult for him to talk. He notes some associated nausea with the pain, but no vomiting. He denies any numbness, tingling, or paresthesia in this left lower leg, and his pain is a 10 out of 10. He denies any prior history of a frank dislocation, but has had some anterior knee pain in the past.

Social History

This 11-year-old male plays soccer for a town recreational league, and has two older brothers. He lives at home with his parents and siblings.

CLINICAL PEARL

Radiographs should be obtained when possible both before and after a patellar dislocation has occurred. The possibility for osteochondral fracture is possible during either dislocation or the reduction of the dislocation, and determining the root cause and comorbidity is important for patient care. The incidence of osteochondral fracture is approximately 30% of all patellar dislocations (Chotel, Bernard, & Raux, 2014).

Physical Assessment

The patient is an 11-year-old male who is in acute distress; it is difficult for him to either sit or lie still or to speak in full sentences. He is 5'4" and weighs 141 lb. He is unable to weight bear. His left lower extremity is externally rotated at the hip, and the knee is flexed to 20 degrees. There is obvious deformity over the patella. A moderate joint effusion is present and noted with inspection and palpation. He is unwilling to move his knee through any range of motion. There is good color, motion, and sensation distal to the knee.

Diagnostic Evaluations

A radiograph was obtained. While moving to the x-ray table, the patella spontaneously reduced. X-rays revealed no facture or current dislocation; a shallow trochlear groove was demonstrated (see Figure 6.3).

CLINICAL PEARL

Often, the inadvertent movement of positioning the leg for an x-ray evaluation will result in a spontaneous reduction of the dislocation. If this does not occur, and the dislocation is recent, the nurse practitioner would attempt reduction with encouraging relaxation with deep breathing and distraction, and gentle medial pressure on the patella to reduce the dislocation. Should this not occur with the first attempt, medication for sedation is indicated.

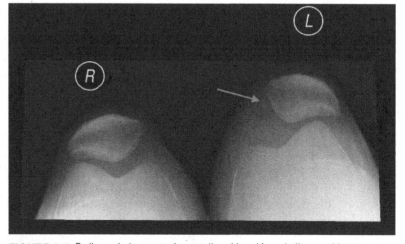

FIGURE 6.3 Radiograph demonstrating patella subluxed in a shallow trochlear groove.

Diagnosis

Patellar dislocation and reduction.

Interventions

The patient was placed into a patellar stabilizing brace and given instructions on decreasing the inflammation; follow-up was recommended for 2 weeks. If a patellar stabilizing brace is not available, then a knee immobilizer is sufficient.

Patient Education

Recommended strategies to teach the patient to decrease inflammation include rest, icing for 20 minutes at least three times a day, and elevating above the heart. Rehabilitation is necessary, with formal physical therapy recommended with a typical frequency and duration of two to three times a week for 6 weeks.

Follow-Up Evaluation

At the initial 2-week follow-up visit, assess the patient for reduction of inflammation, and for readiness for physical therapy. If the effusion and discomfort has subsided, begin physical therapy. The subsequent follow-up visit is recommended at the 6-week postinjury mark. At this visit, information from the physical therapist will be helpful in determining the need for the patient to have follow-up with an orthopedic surgeon for further evaluation, or in determining if the patient has made satisfactory progress and is able to ambulate without a limp or feelings of instability.

REFERENCES

Chotel F., Bernard, J., & Raux, S. (2014). Patellar instability in children and adolescents. *Orthopaedics & Traumatology: Surgery & Research, 100*(1), S125–S137.

Koh, J. L., & Stewart, C. (2014). Patellar instability. *Clinics in Sports Medicine, 33*(3), 461–476.

Case Study 6.4: Chronic Osteoarthritis

Karen M. Myrick

SETTING: ORTHOPEDIC URGENT CARE

Definition and Incidence

Osteoarthritis is characterized by degeneration of the joint cartilage and underlying bone, and patients typically present with joint pain with weight-bearing activities (Kraus, Blanco, Englund, Karsdal, & Lohmander, 2015). Osteoarthritis affects up to 23% of the population (Ma, Chan, & Carruthers, 2014).

Patient

Patient presents with the chief complaint of right "knee pain." He describes a history of an insidious onset of pain that is exacerbated with weight bearing or long periods of sitting with the knee in a flexed position. He has tried both ice and heat, which have not helped much at all. He has also tried acetaminophen 650 mg twice a day, and ibuprofen 800 mg three times a day with minimal relief. He has applied ice and an over-the-counter heat patch during the day, and this seems to help slightly, along with the over-the-counter compression sleeve that he has used for the past month and a half. At this point, he feels that his discomfort is interfering with his ability to play golf and interact with his grandchildren, getting up and down on the floor to play with them.

Social History

This 67-year-old male is a retired engineer, and lives at home with his wife in a ranch-style condominium. He is active with walking 1 to 2 miles a day for exercise, and playing golf.

Physical Assessment

The patient is a 67-year-old male who is in no acute distress; he ambulates without an antalgic gait, but as he rises from a seated position, he is slow and cautious about the first couple of steps. He is 6'1" and weighs 210 lb. On inspection, there is a mild joint effusion, and no open cuts or abrasions in the right knee. With palpation, there are mild crepitations in the tibiofemoral and patellafemoral joint. There is mild tenderness with palpation of the medial and lateral joint lines, both anteriorly and posteriorly. Range of motion in the knee is from 0 to 135, and there is a negative flexion pinch and no ligamentous laxity appreciated. Quadriceps and hamstring strength are 5 out of 5. There are no focal neurological deficits in the right lower extremity.

Diagnostic Evaluations

Radiographs were obtained. Anterior–posterior and lateral views demonstrate medial joint space narrowing, mild subchondral sclerosis, and small osteophytes in the medial compartment of the right knee (see Figure 6.4).

Diagnosis

Osteoarthritis, right knee.

Interventions

The patient was encouraged to work on weight loss, keeping activity moderate, and to limit long periods of sitting with a flexed knee position. He is given a prescription for formal physical therapy, to work on lower extremity and core strengthening.

Patient Education

Importantly, discuss the treatment options with the patient for conservative management, and the step-wise process that is typical for osteoarthritis. Typically, a trial of lifestyle modifications is recommended.

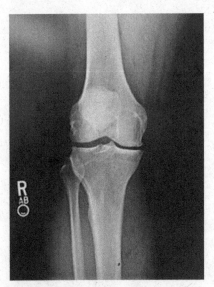

FIGURE 6.4 Radiograph of the knee demonstrating arthritis with medial joint space narrowing, osteophytes, and subchondral sclerosis.

These modifications include weight loss, increasing moderate activity, and strengthening of the lower extremity and core muscles. The potential for corticosteroid intra-articular injections is discussed, along with the potential for hyaluronic acid injections. If theses conservative measures fail, referral to an orthopedic surgeon is recommended.

Follow-Up Evaluation

Follow-up evaluation at the 6-week mark revealed that the patient was experiencing some decrease in his discomfort. At this point, he was not considering injections of corticosteroids or hyaluronic acid. A 6-month follow-up visit is recommended to assess the patient's symptoms at that time.

REFERENCES

Kraus, V. B., Blanco, F. J., Englund, M., Karsdal, M. A., & Lohmander, L. S. (2015). Call for standardized definitions of osteoarthritis and risk stratification for clinical trials and clinical use. *Osteoarthritis & Cartilage, 23*(8), 1233–1241. doi:10.1016/j.joca.2015.03.036

Ma, V. Y., Chan, L., & Carruthers, K. J. (2014). Incidence, prevalence, costs, and impact on disability of common conditions requiring rehabilitation in the United States: Stroke, spinal cord injury, traumatic brain injury, multiple sclerosis, osteoarthritis, rheumatoid arthritis, limb loss. *Archives of Physical Medicine & Rehabilitation, 95*(5), 986.e1–995.e1. doi:10.1016/j.apmr.2013.10.032

Case Study 6.5: Chronic Patellafemoral Pain

Karen M. Myrick

SETTING: PRIMARY CARE

Definition and Incidence

Patellofemoral pain syndrome (PFPS) is commonly a complaint of overuse, and defined as discomfort in the patellofemoral region or anterior knee. PFPS is the most common of acute knee pain seen by primary care providers, orthopedics, and sports medicine specialists (Ho, Hu, Colletti, & Powers, 2014).

Patient

Patient presents with the chief complaint of right "knee pain." She describes a history of the insidious onset of pain in the anterior right knee. Pain seems to be worse with stair climbing, and achy in quality. She describes a feeling that the kneecap might move out of place at times. She has recently been starting on her soccer team and playing for longer periods during games. She has tried Motrin, 200 mg that has helped a little. There are no other myalgias or arthralgias.

Social History

This 14-year-old female is a freshman in high school, and plays on the travel soccer team in her town and on her high school team as well. She lives at home with her two parents and a younger brother.

> ### CLINICAL PEARL
>
> PFPS is more common in the female than male population and more common in the adolescent years (Boling, Padua, & Marshall, 2010).

Physical Assessment

The patient is a 14-year-old female who is in no acute distress. She is 5'4" and weighs 142 lb. Her gait is not antalgic, and she walks with a slight internal rotation to the lower extremities. With palpation, there is no joint effusion or localized warmth. Range of motion in the knee is from 0 to 135 with a negative flexion pinch. Quadriceps and hamstring strength are 5 out of 5 and equal to the contralateral leg, but the vastus medialis is poorly defined. There is a positive patellafemoral compression test, and a negative apprehension test. There are no focal neurological deficits in the left lower extremity.

> **CLINICAL PEARL**
>
> Be sure to evaluate the patient's feet. Frequently, pes planus, or flat foot-edness is concurrent with PFPS.

Diagnostic Evaluations

A radiograph was not obtained, due to the lack of yield on information that would be likely in this patient.

Diagnosis

Patellafemoral pain syndrome.

Interventions

The patient was encouraged to begin a course of physical therapy, with the recommended frequency of two to three times a week for 6 weeks. She was educated on the natural course of PFPS, the importance of physical therapy, and continuation of the exercises.

Patient Education

It is important for the patient to be educated on the factor that overuse has in the process of PFPS, and how the imbalance of the musculature of the lower extremities may influence the syndrome and also allow for the avoidance of symptoms. Keeping the iliotibial band flexible with proficient stretching and keeping the vastus medialis strong are key to symptom alleviation.

Follow-Up Evaluation

Patient returns after a 6-week course of physical therapy, at which time her symptoms have decreased significantly. She will progress to a home exercise program, and follow up on an as-needed basis.

REFERENCES

Boling, M., Padua, D., & Marshall, S. (2010). Gender differences in the incidence and prevalence of patellofemoral pain syndrome. *Scandinavian Journal of Medicine and Science in Sports, 20*(5), 725–730.

Ho, K., Hu, H. H., Colletti, P. M., & Powers, C. M. (2014). Running-induced patellofemoral pain fluctuates with changes in patella water content. *European Journal of Sport Science, 14*(6), 628–634. doi:10.1080/17461391.2013.862872

Case Study 6.6: Chronic Patellar Tendinitis

Karen M. Myrick

SETTING: PRIMARY CARE

Definition and Incidence

Chronic patellar tendinitis is characterized by pain and tenderness in the anterior knee, at the patellar tendon, and typically the inferior pole of the patella (Brockmeyer, Diehl, Schmitt, Dieter, & Lorbach, 2015).

Patient

Patient presents with the chief complaint of left "knee pain." He describes a history of increasing activity recently with the onset of the basketball season. New this year, he is in the starting lineup on his university's team. He has been training with the team, and also on his own, increasing his plyometric exercises in an effort to improve his vertical jump. He describes the discomfort coming on slowly over the past 2 to 3 weeks, and now is at the level of a 6 out of 10 when playing basketball. He does not notice any associated swelling; there is no locking, catching, or giving way; and the pain is not associated with a limp. He tried ibuprofen, 800 mg once or twice, but really did not find this to make a difference in the swelling or discomfort. Applying ice 20 minutes four to five times a day has been beneficial in reducing discomfort, but this causes too much stiffness to try prior to play.

Social History

This 19-year-old male is a sophomore in college. He was recruited to the school to play on a scholarship. He lives 4 hours away from the school he attends.

Physical Assessment

The patient is a 19-year-old male who is in no acute distress, but demonstrates mild discomfort at points of the examination. He is 6'3" and weighs 219 lb. His gait is not antalgic. On inspection, there is no joint effusion, and no open cuts or abrasions. With palpation, there is pain at the proximal part of the patellar tendon and at the inferior patellar pole. The extensor mechanism is intact. Range of motion in the knee is from 0 to 135 degrees and pain free. He has a negative flexion pinch and no ligamentous laxity is appreciated. Quadriceps and hamstring strength are 5 out of 5 and equal bilaterally.

There are no focal neurological deficits in the left lower extremity; he has excellent color, sensation, and movement.

Diagnostic Evaluations

A radiograph was not obtained, due to the lack of yield on information that would be likely in this patient.

Diagnosis

Patellar tendinitis.

Interventions

The patient was encouraged to decrease activity and to have a modified rest period for the next 3 weeks, and return for follow-up. Modified rest was described as rest from jumping activities in particular. Ice, 20 minutes three times a day, was recommended.

Patient Education

Educating the patient about improving his flexibility, especially the quadriceps in order to help decrease the pull of the patellar tendon on the insertion site, is beneficial to decrease recurrence, and prevent future injuries. Discussing the role of overtraining or overuse is also important with any tendinitis problem.

Follow-Up Evaluation

At the follow-up visit, the patient reported that his pain had decreased to a 1 out of 10. Physical therapy was ordered to work on eccentric training and core strengthening was ordered. A repeat evaluation in 6 weeks revealed that the patient was pain free and wanting to get back to full physical activity.

REFERENCE

Brockmeyer, M., Diehl, N., Schmitt, C., Dieter, K. M., & Lorbach, O. (2015). Results of surgical treatment of chronic patellar tendinosis (Jumper's Knee): A systematic review of the literature. *Arthroscopy: Journal of Arthroscopy & Related Surgery, 31*(12), 2424.e3–2429.e3. doi:10.1016/j.arthro.2015.06.010

CHAPTER 7

Ankle

Case Study 7.1: Acute Ankle Fracture

Karen M. Myrick

SETTING: URGENT CARE

Definition and Incidence

Ankle fractures are common, and occur at an annual incidence of one in every 800 people (Mehta, Rees, Cutler, & Mangwani, 2014). Ankle fractures occur across the life span and with a variety of mechanisms of injury.

Patient

Patient presents with the chief complaint of right ankle pain. She describes a history of walking her dog when she stepped into a hole that she was not aware of. She twisted her ankle, and felt pain immediately. She was not able to ambulate home, and used her cell phone to call her husband who came to pick her up. She has not been able to bear weight on the ankle since the injury, and has pain that is a 7 out of 10. She notices swelling and bruising over the lateral ankle. There is no associated numbness or tingling, and pain is less with ice that she placed on her ankle on her way to the clinic.

Social History

This 37-year-old female is a stay-at-home mother who has a small business in consulting for fitness. She has three children: twin girls aged 4, and a 5-year-old son who is in kindergarten this year.

Physical Assessment

The patient is a 37-year-old female who is in no acute distress, but demonstrates hesitancy and some discomfort throughout the physical examination. She is 5'4" and weighs 132 lb. She is unable to weight bear in the clinic, and hops onto the examining table for assessment. On inspection, there is a moderate amount of swelling over the lateral ankle, and ecchymosis in a somewhat dependent pattern as well. The skin is intact without tenting or open cuts or abrasions. With palpation, she has bony tenderness that begins 6 cm above the malleolus, and is tender to the lateral malleolus with palpation. She has no tenderness with medial palpation, including over the deltoid ligament. Dorsalis pedis and posterior tibialis pulses were strong and intact. She is hesitant to perform range of motion (ROM) in the ankle, but is able to move all of her toes, and to demonstrate approximately 10 degrees of ankle dorsiflexion and plantar flexion. There are no focal neurological deficits in the left lower extremity, and good color throughout.

> ### CLINICAL PEARL
>
> The presence of any medial injury determines the stability of fractures of the medial malleolus (Goost et al., 2014).

Diagnostic Evaluations

Radiographs were obtained, including an anterioposterior, lateral, and mortise view. The x-ray demonstrated a fracture of the distal fibula of the right ankle (see Figure 7.1). The ankle mortise is intact and anatomically aligned, as is seen on the mortise view, Figure 7.2.

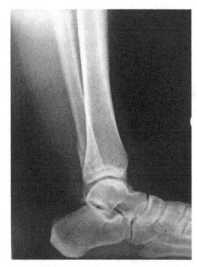

FIGURE 7.1 Radiograph demonstrating a fracture of the distal fibula.

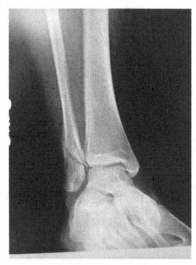

FIGURE 7.2 Radiograph of the ankle, mortise view, demonstrating the intact mortise without widening.

Diagnosis

Fractured fibula, right ankle.

Interventions

The patient was placed into a posterior and U-splint and given crutches. She was instructed to be nonweight bearing until her follow-up visit, and a follow-up visit was made for 8 days later. She was instructed to move her toes frequently, ice 20 minutes several times a day, and elevate above the level of the heart.

Patient Education

Teach the patient that a large majority of pain from the injury will be due to inflammation. It is important to practice modalities that will decrease and keep inflammation at bay to help with the healing process and to keep the discomfort under control.

Follow-Up Evaluation

This patient followed up in 8 days and was placed into a walking boot. She was instructed to return in 2 weeks for x-ray evaluation. She returned at the 2-week time point, and the radiographic evaluation demonstrated early callus formation and stability to the fracture. She was allowed to weight bear for the next 2 weeks, and returned for x-rays that demonstrated healing of the fracture. She was placed into a stirrup splint and told to begin physical therapy and return at the 6-week mark. At the 6-week mark, she was ambulatory without pain, had occasional swelling at the end of the day, and was ready to return to full activities.

REFERENCES

Goost, H., Wimmer, M. D., Barg, A., Kabir, K., Valderrabano, V., & Burger, C. (2014). Fractures of the ankle joint. *Deutsches Aerzteblatt International, 111*(21), 377–388. doi:10.3238/arztebl.2014.0377

Mehta, S., Rees, K., Cutler, L., & Mangwani, J. (2014). Understanding risks and complications in the management of ankle fractures. *Indian Journal of Orthopaedics* [serial online], *48*(5), 445–452.

Case Study 7.2: Acute Achilles Tendon Rupture

Phoebe M. Heffron

SETTING: ORTHOPEDIC URGENT CARE

Definition and Incidence

The Achilles tendon is a long fibrous tissue in the posterior lower leg that attaches distally to the calcaneus and proximally to the gastrocnemius and soleus muscles. Achilles tendon ruptures have increased more than tenfold over the past several decades from 2.1 in 100,000 to 21.5 in 100,000 (Lantto, Heikkinen, Flinkkilä, Ohtonen, & Leppilahti, 2015).

Patient

Patient presents to orthopedic urgent care, complaining of pain in the back of his left lower leg. He states, "I was playing basketball two nights ago in my men's recreation league game. I drove down the lane to shoot a layup and heard a pop; it felt like someone hit me in the back of the leg with a baseball bat. I immediately crumpled to the floor in pain." The patient states that his teammates helped him up and assisted him to the sidelines—he was able to bear some weight but it was very painful. Once he got to the sidelines, he applied ice immediately. Over the course of the past 36 hours, he has noticed some bruising and swelling. He has continued to ice intermittently. He has taken ibuprofen 600 mg twice a day and says, "It's still sore but not quite as painful." He has an old elastic bandage at home that he has been wearing. He has continued to go to work, play with his children, and help cook and clean but feels like his gait is off. He has not attempted to go back to the gym since the injury.

Social History

This 42-year-old man is a father of two young boys. He was away on business for the past 2 weeks and was excited to get back home to his weekly basketball game. He has had ankle problems before and is worried this is more serious than his previous sprained ankles. He is frustrated by the possibility of a lengthy recovery and is worried about how he will manage shoveling and snow-blowing duties this winter.

CLINICAL PEARL

Achilles tendon injuries are most often seen in men in their 40s and 50s (Pedowitz & Kirwan, 2013).

Physical Assessment

The patient is a 42-year-old male who stands 5'11" tall and weighs 170 lb. He sits on the exam table in no acute distress. He walks on his tiptoes in obvious discomfort. His lower calf has moderate swelling and bruising. The left foot is of normal temperature and color, has a capillary refill of less than 3 seconds, and demonstrates a 2+ posterior tibial pulse. When lying prone with feet hanging off the table, the left foot lies in decreased plantar flexion compared with the right side. Palpation shows notable step off in the Achilles tendon about 5 cm superior to the calcaneus. The Thompson test is positive.

Diagnostic Evaluations

An MRI may be obtained in cases of diagnostic uncertainty; often, however, the diagnosis is clear and additional imaging can delay treatment. An x-ray is unlikely to aid in the diagnosis.

Diagnosis

Achilles tendon rupture.

Intervention

The nurse practitioner provides the patient with a set of crutches, a posterior splint, and advice to be nonweight bearing. The splint has a slight equinus position (plantar flexion) to keep the tendon lengthened and as approximated as possible. He is scheduled to see an orthopedic surgeon today to discuss the possibility of surgical intervention.

Patient Education

As a nurse practitioner, you must be able to educate the patient on treatment options including surgical versus nonsurgical treatment, the recovery time, and benefits and adverse outcomes associated with the different treatment modalities.

Follow-Up Evaluation

As it is possible that this patient will have a surgical intervention, the nurse practitioner may not have the opportunity to follow up directly unless working in a setting where nurses collaborate with the orthopedic surgeon. In such a case, the nurse practitioner may write a prescription for pain medication and physical therapy and may see the patient postoperatively. It is even possible that the nurse practitioner will assist the orthopedist during surgery. If the patient opts for nonsurgical rehabilitation, the nurse practitioner working in orthopedics may also have the opportunity to prescribe a course of physical therapy. For a nurse practitioner in a primary care setting, he or she may not see this patient again for this particular injury but will likely encounter other patients with Achilles tendon injuries during the time in practice. It is imperative that the nurse practitioner understands that prompt treatment is essential for optimal patient outcomes, particularly if the patient elects to have surgery. The nurse practitioner in primary care may also help this patient with paperwork needed to apply for short-term disability through his employer.

REFERENCES

Lantto, I., Heikkinen, J., Flinkkilä, T., Ohtonen, P., & Leppilahti, J. (2015) Epidemiology of Achilless tendon ruptures: Increasing incidence over a 33-year period. *Scandinavian Journal of Medicine & Science in Sports, 25,* e133–e138. doi:10.1111/sms.12253

Pedowitz, D., & Kirwan, G. (2013). Achilles tendon ruptures. *Current Reviews in Musculoskeletal Medicine, 6*(4), 285–293. doi:10.1007/s12178-013-9185-8

Case Study 7.3: Acute Peroneal Tendon Dislocation

Karen M. Myrick

SETTING: ACUTE CARE

Definition and Incidence

Peroneal tendon subluxations or dislocations are often mistaken as simple ankle sprains, and may go undiagnosed (Espinosa & Maurer, 2015). The peroneal tendons are held in the fibular groove by the superior peroneal retinaculum, which can be torn with forceful ankle dorsiflexion and eversion injuries (Espinosa & Maurer, 2015).

Patient

A 17-year-old patient presents to the urgent care with the chief complaint of ankle pain. Just 2 hours prior to presentation, she reports running on the soc-cer field when she unexpectedly stepped into a hole in the turf. She reports that she felt a pop in the ankle, and fell to the ground. She was unable to weight bear initially, and was helped to the sidelines by a teammate and her coach. She placed ice on the ankle immediately, and elevated it as well. After the game, she was able to minimally weight bear with an antalgic gait to the car with her parents and came right to the urgent care clinic for evaluation. Pain is worse when the limb is kept dependent; it is better with elevation. She describes the pain as 6 out of 10 without pressure; when bearing weight, the pain is 8 out of 10. She denies any numbness or tingling of the lower leg.

Social History

This 17-year-old female is a high school junior, and plays with a travel soccer team, as well as with her high school team.

CLINICAL PEARL

Dislocated peroneal tendons are often misdiagnosed as lateral ankle sprains, and occur in approximately 0.3% to 0.5% of traumatic injuries to the ankle (Espinosa & Maurer, 2015).

Physical Assessment

The patient is a 17-year-old female who stands 5'5" tall and weighs 130 lb. She is in no acute distress, but mild discomfort. She is able to weight bear, but has an antalgic gait, favoring the left side. She has mild swelling just posterior to the lateral malleolus on the left. There is no boney point tenderness over the malleolus or distal fibula. Ankle ROM is limited in all planes due to pain. With special testing, an anterior drawer test and talar tilt test are negative, without increased translation compared to the contralateral side. With peroneal ligament testing, a palpable snap is exhibited when the patient everts the ankle against resistance. This is considered a positive test.

Diagnostic Evaluations

Ankle radiographs are not performed, as the patient has no bony tenderness and can weight bear. An ultrasound is performed which demonstrates peroneal dislocation from the fibular groove.

> ### CLINICAL PEARL
>
> Ultrasonography is the imaging method of choice, as peroneal subluxation may not always be visible on static images as with an MRI (Neustadter, Raikin, & Nazarian, 2004).

Diagnosis

Acute peroneal tendon subluxation.

Intervention

A walking boot is placed for the patient's comfort and to provide stability. Recommendations for rest, ice, and elevation are provided. She is scheduled in follow-up for consultation to see an orthopedic surgeon next week.

Patient Education

Educate the patient on the treatment options including surgical versus nonsurgical treatment, the recovery time, and benefits and adverse outcomes associated with the different treatment modalities.

Follow-Up Evaluation

If the patient chooses nonoperative treatment, and agrees to modify her activity, follow-up would be recommended at the 6-week mark after a trial of physical therapy. With surgical consultation, it is possible that the nurse practitioner may not follow-up directly with the patient, but may provide preoperative education for the patient to assist with expectations and recovery. If the nurse practitioner is in a setting working collaboratively with an orthopedic surgeon, he or she may perform the preoperative and postoperative care of the patient, and may also be in a position to first assist in the operating room for the surgical repair of the retinaculum.

REFERENCES

Espinosa, N., & Maurer, M. A. (2015). Peroneal tendon dislocation. *European Journal of Trauma & Emergency Surgery, 41*(6), 631–637. doi:10.1007/s00068-015-0590-0

Neustadter, J., Raikin, S. M., & Nazarian, L. N. (2004). Dynamic sonographic evaluation of peroneal tendon subluxation. *American Journal of Roentgenology, 183*(4), 985–988. doi:0361–803X/04/1834-985

Case Study 7.4: Chronic Ankle Instability

Kevin Fitzsimmons

SETTING: SPORTS MEDICINE CLINIC

Definition and Incidence

In the United States, an estimated 2 million ankle sprains occur each year. Ankle injuries are the most common sports-related injury, with some estimates attributing lateral ankle sprain to over 40% of all sports-related injuries (Ferran & Maffuli, 2006). It is estimated that approximately 60% to 80% of these ankle sprains resolve with conservative measures such as rest, ice, anti-inflammatory medication, temporary bracing, and physical therapy (Ferran & Maffuli, 2006; Waterman, Belmont, Cameron, DeBerardino, & Owens, 2010). However, current literature suggests that up to 20% of the remaining ankle sprains do not completely resolve and chronic ankle instability persists (Ferran & Maffuli, 2006; Waterman et al., 2010). The lateral ankle ligaments are most commonly injured in this order from anterior to posterior: anterior talofibular ligament (ATFL), calcaneofibular ligament (CFL), and posterior talofibular ligament (PTFL) (Beynnon, Murphy, & Alosa, 2002; Kaminski, 2013).

Patient

The patient is a 15-year-old female who first presented to sports medicine clinic 9 weeks after suffering an acute right lateral ankle sprain during lacrosse activities. She reports cutting to change direction, and describes an inversion type mechanism with immediate lateral ankle pain and swelling. She denied medial ankle pain and knee pain. She was unable to ambulate off the field without assistance. Rest, ice, and anti-inflammatory medication were implemented initially. Nonweight-bearing x-rays were performed of her right ankle at the first sports medicine clinic visit at 4 days postinjury, and were negative for fracture, or widening of the mortise. The patient was placed in a walking boot, and prescribed physical therapy. The patient reports her symptoms improved at rest over the course of the first 4 weeks, but reported continued pain and "giving way" episodes even when braced as she attempted to return to physical activity at 6 to 8 weeks postinjury. She was then referred to further evaluation.

Social History

The patient is a 15-year-old female, entering her sophomore year of high school. This is her first ankle sprain, and most severe injury she has sustained at this time. She has an excellent support system with mother and father at home as well as a younger sibling. She demonstrates excellent coping skills with discussion of the options both nonoperative and operative.

CLINICAL PEARL

When concerned for chronic ankle instability, frequently stress radiographs are obtained. If pain occurs during the stress radiographs, the evaluation is considered invalid as the presence of muscle spasm from pain can reduce the sensitivity of exam. Stress radiographs must be performed bilaterally for comparison.

Physical Assessment

This 15-year-old female appears to be well and in no acute distress. Left ankle exam reveals mild lateral ankle swelling, without erythema or ecchymosis. No tenderness to palpation of the lateral malleolus, medial malleolus, deltoid ligament, distal tibiofibular joint, and proximal fibula. She has full ROM and strength in all planes compared bilaterally. The patient is neurovascularly intact distally with symmetric sensation along the tibial, superficial, and deep peroneal nerve. A positive and pain-free anterior drawer and talar tilt for laxity is demonstrated. She has a negative Kleiger test and forefoot squeeze test.

Diagnostic Evaluations

Stress x-rays (Figures 7.3 and 7.4) of the right ankle demonstrate significant talar tilt and anterior talar translation compared to the contralateral side (Figures 7.5 and 7.6).

Diagnosis

Right chronic ankle instability.

Interventions

There is a discussion of risks, benefits, and alternatives regarding continued conservative management versus operative intervention. Due to her continued instability and positive stress radiographs, the patient and her family chose to move forward with operative treatment consisting of right

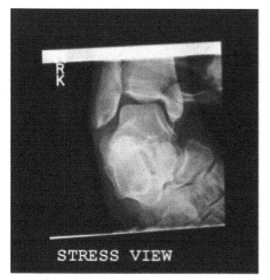

FIGURE 7.3 AP view stress radiograph of the right (involved/injured) ankle demonstrating increased widening of lateral aspect of mortise (talar tilt).

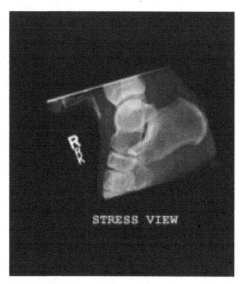

FIGURE 7.4 Lateral view stress radiograph of the right (involved/injured) ankle demonstrating increased anterior displacement of talus.

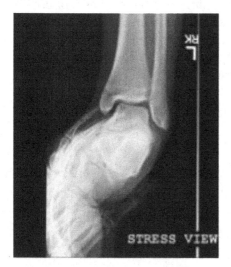

FIGURE 7.5 AP view stress radiograph of the left (uninvolved/uninjured) ankle demonstrating slight widening of lateral aspect of mortise when compared to involved (right ankle stress radiograph).

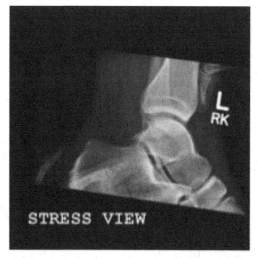

FIGURE 7.6 Lateral view stress radiograph of the left (uninvolved/uninjured) ankle demonstrating less anterior translation of the talus compared to involved (right ankle stress radiograph).

ankle arthroscopy, with Brostrom-Gould lateral ankle ligament repair. This procedure involves removing abnormal or injured ligamentous tissue and suturing the injured ligaments, the ATFL, and CFL to create scar tissue and eventually improve stability of the ankle joint.

Patient Education

Educate the patient that after lateral ankle ligament repair, there is a low rate of recurrent instability and pain. However, if recurrent instability were to occur, a formal ligament reconstruction utilizing tendon autograft can be performed if initial conservative management fails.

Follow-Up Evaluation

After surgery, the right lower leg was immobilized in a cast for 6 weeks, and then physical therapy was performed for approximately 6 months afterward. She reported no pain or episodes of "giving way," painful crepitance, or recurrent swelling at 7 months postoperatively. She was cleared to return to sports at the 7-month mark postoperatively and has been doing well since. No recurrent ankle instability events have been reported as of her 1-year postoperative follow-up.

REFERENCES

Beynnon, B. D., Murphy, D. F., & Alosa, D. M. (2002). Predictive factors for lateral ankle sprains: A literature review. *Journal of Athletic Training (National Athletic Trainers' Association)*, 37(4), 376–380.

Ferran, N. A., & Maffuli, N. (2006). Epidemiology of sprains of the lateral ankle ligament complex. *Foot Ankle Clinics*, 11(3), 659–662.

Kaminski, T. W., Hertel, J., Amendola, N., Docherty, C. L., Dolan, M. G., Ty Hopkins, J., . . . Richie, D. (2013). National Athletic Trainers' Association position statement: Conservative management and prevention of ankle sprains in athletes. *Journal of Athletic Training*, 48(4), 528–545. doi:10.4085/1062-6050-48.4.02

Waterman, B. R., Belmont, Jr., P. J., Cameron, K. L., DeBerardino, T. M., & Owens, B. D. (2010). Epidemiology of ankle sprain at the United States Military Academy. *American Journal of Sports Medicine*, 38(4), 797–803.

Case Study 7.5: Chronic Ankle Pain (talar osteochondral defect)

Scott A. Myrick

SETTING: PRIMARY CARE

Definition and Incidence

Osteochondral defects (OCDs) of the talus are increasingly recognized common injuries and may occur in up to 50% of ankle sprains and fractures (Bisicchia, Rosso, & Amendola, 2014). Repetitive trauma to the ankle joint can damage not only the surrounding ankle ligaments, but also potentially damage the articular cartilage surfaces.

Patient

A 20-year-old male basketball player comes to the office with a complaint of consistent right ankle pain. This pain is typically nonexistent upon awaking, gets progressively worse throughout the day, and is much worse with activity. Running and jumping make a specific, marked increase in his pain. In his past, the only injuries he's suffered surround recurring ankle sprains on his right leg. He mentions he has never had a fracture, however, but does feel "clunking" in his ankle, which is sometimes painful.

While a good-natured young man, he was clearly frustrated with a persistent pain keeping him from practicing some days. Besides being very active on the basketball court, the patient usually participates in a regular strength and conditioning program. As of late, his ankle pain has prevented him from doing even this.

Social History

The patient has been playing basketball since he was around 7 years old. Having been very active most of his life, he does not smoke and drinks only occasionally.

CLINICAL PEARL

For ankle injuries, balance and proprioceptive training can be a very important piece of both injury prevention and injury rehabilitation. This typically includes one-leg training, stance training, and exercises that focus on the hip musculature and can help control the lower leg.

Physical Assessment

The patient presents today in some distress. He describes a constant aching pain in the anterior area of his ankle mortise. He is muscular at 6'6" and 225 lb. Upon close examination of the ankle itself, some swelling is present. With ROM testing, the patient demonstrates reduced dorsiflexion with apparent stiffness and some discomfort. Plantar flexion and inversion are increased relative to the contralateral uninjured side by roughly 10 degrees. Upon resisted strength testing, the muscles surrounding the ankle joint are generally strong. The one exception is that of resisted eversion; the weakness of the peroneals is consistent with his history of recurrent ankle sprains. Testing of the ligaments reveals increased laxity on anterior drawer test for the ATFL. Also of note is increased laxity of the CFL with inversion.

Diagnostic Evaluations

Radiographs were obtained to look for the presence of any avulsion or bony fragments. A fragment, most likely of articular cartilage, is seen anterior to the talus.

The MRI demonstrated obvious laxity in the ligaments themselves, inflammation and swelling in the anterior ankle around the talus, and some clear damage to the anterior proximal talus itself. Also of note is some damage to the ATFL (Figure 7.7).

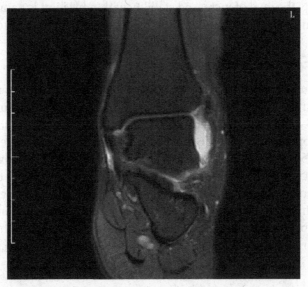

FIGURE 7.7 MRI demonstrating laxity of the ligaments in the ankle and a joint effusion.

Diagnosis

Right ankle osteochondral defect with instability.

Interventions

The patient was educated on the rest, ice, compression, elevation (RICE) treatment of resting his ankle from aggravating movements to include no impact activity. He was instructed on a regimen of nonsteroidal anti-inflammatory drugs (NSAIDs) and icing four to six times daily.

With his rest period from basketball, a prescription of physical therapy was implemented with the goals to reduce his chronic swelling, decrease his pain, and improve his dynamic stability through increased proprioception and strength around his ankle joint.

Follow-up within 3 to 5 weeks was arranged to gauge progress. If there is no resolution in his symptoms and he is unable to return to his desired level of activity, surgical intervention will be considered. This option is described to him along with the implications of surgery and he understands this.

Patient Education

With a rehab regime, the patient must understand his role and the provider must achieve buy-in. When both provider and patient are on the same page, the likelihood of achieving stated goals increases dramatically. Therefore, the patient must understand not to engage in aggravating activity, and be disciplined in the rehab protocol. If this fails, the provider follow-up will dictate the next options.

With the consideration of surgery, the patient must understand the goal. Surely the goal of increased stability within his joint is paramount. With that, add decreased pain and swelling and a graduated return to activity.

Follow-Up Evaluation

Because this injury may require surgical consultation, the nurse practitioner may not follow the patient throughout the entire continuum of care. If the nurse practitioner is in a setting where nurses work collaboratively with an orthopedic surgeon, the nurse may refer the patient if there is no initial progress being made or simply collaborate on the most effective course of treatment. For the primary care nurse practitioner, it is likely the patient would return after rehabilitation has been completed in order to gauge the athlete's readiness to return to his or her sport. This may be done in conjunction and collaboration with the physical therapist and/or athletic trainer. In the case of surgery, the follow-up may be overseen by the surgeon.

REFERENCE

Bisicchia, S., Rosso, F., & Amendola, A. (2014). Talar osteochondral defects: Current techniques. *Operative Techniques in Sports Medicine, 22*(4), 331–338. doi:10.1053/j.otsm.2014.09.006

Case Study 7.6: Chronic Peroneal Tendon Dislocation/Subluxation

Phoebe M. Heffron

SETTING: PRIMARY CARE OFFICE

Definition and Incidence

The peroneal tendons are responsible for eversion of the foot; the peroneus brevis inserts on the lower leg runs posterior to the fibula, and inserts onto the fifth metatarsal; the peroneus longus originates more proximally and runs all the way under the foot to attach to the first metatarsal (see Figure 7.8). These tendons rest in a groove along the back of the fibula and are held in place by the superior peroneal retinaculum. A chronic subluxed peroneal tendon usually results from an acute injury that has healed improperly. The initial injuries often occur in sports with a jumping component. Frequently, other ankle injuries or instabilities occur concurrently (DiGiovanni, Fraga, Cohen, & Shereff, 2000).

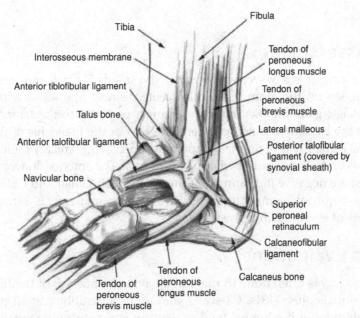

FIGURE 7.8 Anatomy of the lateral ankle, including the peroneal tendons.

Patient

A 37-year-old patient presents to her primary care provider complaining of chronic ankle pain. "I injured my ankle a couple months ago playing soccer when I turned my ankle. I assumed it was just a sprain and tried rest, ice, and wearing a brace, but it's still pretty tender. Every once in a while, if I step on uneven ground or something, I have a sudden sharp pain and sometimes hear a snapping sound. It usually returns to the constant dull ache in a short period of time. I've tried taking anti-inflammatory medication but that doesn't give me much relief." She reports that there was some initial swelling and bruising and though the bruising has gone away, she still has some swelling over the lateral ankle. She does acknowledge having occasional episodes of instability.

Social History

This 37-year-old woman is a stay-at-home mother to 15-month-old boy–girl twins. Her husband works long hours and she has no family nearby. Her twins go to day care two mornings a week from 9 to 12 but are primarily in her care. She has been able to deal with the pain enough to continue their daily routine but doesn't know how much longer she can continue to do so especially as her twins are becoming more mobile.

> ### CLINICAL PEARL
>
> Subluxed peroneal tendons are often misdiagnosed as lateral ankle sprains.

Physical Assessment

The patient is a 37-year-old female who stands 5'7" tall and weighs 120 lb. She sits on the exam table in no acute distress. She walks with a slightly antalgic gait. She has mild swelling just posterior to the lateral malleolus on the left. There is no point tenderness over the malleolus or distal fibula. The extremity is of normal temperature and color. Capillary refill is less than 3 seconds; the dorsalis pedis pulse is normal. The anterior drawer test and tilt test are negative indicating that the anterior talofibular and CFLs are intact. The peroneal ligament test is positive as the examiner feels a snap when the patient everts against resistance.

Diagnostic Evaluations

An x-ray is often done to rule out an avulsion fracture of the fibula or lateral malleolus. MRIs, CT-scans, and ultrasonography can all be useful in determining if peroneal tendon damage is present; ultrasonography may be the imaging modality of choice because subluxation may not always be visible on static images as with MRI and CT (Neustadter, Raikin, & Nazarian, 2004).

Diagnosis

Chronic peroneal tendon subluxation.

Interventions

The nurse practitioner provides the patient with a compression bandage and advises her simply to be as cautious as possible. She is scheduled to see an orthopedic surgeon next week.

Patient Education

As a nurse practitioner in primary care, you must be able to educate the patient on treatment options including surgical versus nonsurgical treatment, the recovery time, and benefits and adverse outcomes associated with the different treatment modalities. The nurse practitioner should also remind the patient of the importance of proper stretching before participating in athletic activities.

Follow-Up Evaluation

As it is possible that this patient will have a surgical intervention, the nurse practitioner may not have the opportunity to follow up with her directly. However, due to her ongoing relationship with the patient, the nurse practitioner can emphasize the importance of being nonweight bearing following surgery (if surgical intervention is elected) and adhering to the prescribed physical therapy regiment for optimal outcome. It is important for the nurse practitioner to keep this diagnosis in mind for a patient who presents with a previously diagnosed ankle sprain that is not healing with conservative treatment.

REFERENCES

DiGiovanni, B. F., Fraga, C. J., Cohen, B. E., & Shereff, M. J. (2000). Associated injuries found in chronic lateral ankle instability. *Foot & Ankle International, 21*(10), 809–815. doi:10.1177/107110070002101003

Neustadter, J., Raikin, S. M., & Nazarian, L. N. (2004). Dynamic sonographic evaluation of peroneal tendon subluxation. *American Journal of Roentgenology, 183*(4), 985–988. doi:0361–803X/04/1834-985

CHAPTER **8**

Foot

Case Study 8.1: Acute Metatarsal Fracture

Karen M. Myrick

SETTING: ORTHOPEDIC URGENT CARE

Definition and Incidence

Metatarsal fractures are common in both children and adults (Boutefnouchet, Budair, Backshayesh, & Ali, 2014). Special attention needs to be paid to the fifth metatarsal bone, as it is the most commonly injured metatarsal bone, and can have surgical implications for repair (Boutefnouchet et al., 2014).

Patient

Patient presents with the chief complaint of left foot pain. He describes a history of playing baseball at his high school earlier in the day. He states, "I was running down the first base line when I was tagged out. I stepped on first base, landing slightly off to the side. I felt a sharp pain, and I fell to the ground." He was helped off the field by the athletic trainer and another player, stating he was unable to bear weight. He describes the swelling as immediate, and ice was placed. He watched the end of the game and presents for evaluation. Discomfort is well located in the left foot and moderate, rated as a 6 out of 10. Pain is worse with weight bearing, and associated with a significant limp, favoring the left leg, when attempted.

Social History

This 19-year-old male is in his senior year of high school, and he plans on playing at an intramural level in college.

> ### CLINICAL PEARL
>
> Avulsion fractures are common in the skeletally immature patient with separation at the apophysis as the most frequent injury (Mehlhorn, Zwingmann, Hirschmüller, Südkamp, & Schmal, 2014). An avulsion fracture is commonly treated in a short-leg walking cast for 3 weeks.

Physical Assessment

The patient is a 19-year-old male who is in no acute distress, but demonstrates hesitancy and some discomfort throughout the physical examination. He is 6'3" and weighs 203 lb. His gait is antalgic, demonstrating a shortened stance phase on the left, and pain with any pressure on the left foot. On inspection, there is a moderate joint effusion and no open cuts or abrasions. With palpation, there is bony point tenderness over the midshaft of the fifth metatarsal on the left foot. Range of motion in the left ankle is full and pain free. There are no focal neurological deficits in the left lower extremity.

Diagnostic Evaluations

A radiograph was obtained and demonstrates a midshaft metatarsal fracture on the left foot (see Figure 8.1).

Diagnosis

Midshaft metatarsal fracture left foot.

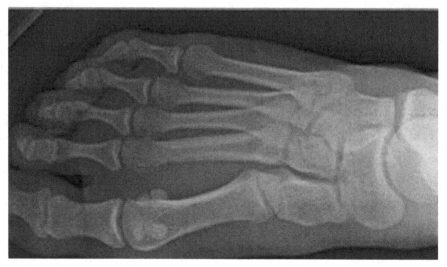

FIGURE 8.1 Fracture of the proximal fifth metatarsal.

Interventions

The patient was placed into a posterior splint, and provided crutches. He was instructed to maintain a nonweight-bearing status until he follows up in 7 to 10 days.

Patient Education

Educate the patient and his family to avoid activity, especially weight bearing, until they follow up for repeat x-rays and definitive management.

Follow-Up Evaluation

The patient was seen in follow-up at 8 days. At that point, his radiographs were repeated, and they demonstrated no change in alignment of the fracture, with fragments well approximated. A firm, supportive shoe was placed and used for the next 4 weeks. And the patient progressively added weight bearing until full within 1 week out from this visit. Four weeks later, radiographs were obtained and demonstrated good healing of the fracture with callus formation, and the patient was provided a prescription for physical therapy at a rate of two to three times a week for the next 4 to 6 weeks with progression back to activity and a home exercise program.

REFERENCES

Boutefnouchet, T., Budair, B., Backshayesh, P., & Ali, S. A. (2014). Metatarsal fractures: A review and current concepts. *Trauma, 16*(3), 147–163. doi:10.1177/1460408614525738

Mehlhorn, A. T., Zwingmann, J., Hirschmüller, A., Südkamp, N. P., & Schmal, H. (2014). Radiographic classification for fractures of the fifth metatarsal base. *Skeletal Radiology, 43*(4), 467–474. doi:10.1007/s00256-013-1810-5

Case Study 8.2: Acute Lisfranc Dislocation

Vinayak M. Sathe, Teja Karukonda, and Daniel Witmer

SETTING: OUTPATIENT CLINIC FOLLOW-UP FROM URGENT CARE CENTER

Definition and Incidence

The Lisfranc complex in the midfoot is an intricate interaction between the first and second metatarsals, the medial and middle cuneiforms, and the ligamentous supports that traverse these joints (Seybold & Coetzee, 2015). High-energy mechanisms of injury or trauma and low-energy injuries in the athlete are the most common mechanisms of injury (Seybold & Coetzee, 2015).

Patient

A 50-year-old female patient presents with right foot pain and swelling of several weeks' duration. It began when she sustained a fall while ambulating; however, she could not recall the exact position of her right foot at the time of the injury. She immediately noticed significant pain, swelling, and bruising over the dorsum of her right foot. She initially presented to an urgent care clinic and was advised that her injury was a benign soft tissue injury and that she could remain weight bearing as tolerated on the right lower extremity in a walking boot with crutches. Over the next 2 weeks, the patient's swelling and ecchymosis partially improved; however, she continued to experience significant pain aggravated by weight bearing and activity as well as persistent swelling at the end of the day. Her pain was localized over the dorsum of the right midfoot and was unresponsive to anti-inflammatory medications or pain relievers. She felt relief when she was not bearing weight on the right foot. In addition, she reported mild numbness over the dorsum of the foot. She denied any other associated symptoms including fevers, chills, or any other musculoskeletal pain or weakness.

Social History

Patient is a college professor at a local community college. She is married and has two adult children.

Physical Assessment

The patient was in no acute distress. She had normal standing alignment with an antalgic gait favoring the left lower extremity. She avoided full weight bearing on the right lower extremity on gait analysis. On focused assessment of her right lower extremity, she was found to have significant swelling and ecchymosis over the dorsum of her right midfoot as well as plantar ecchymosis in the arch of the foot. Her skin was intact with no abrasions or lacerations. She had tenderness to palpation localized over the bases of the first and second metatarsals as well as over the medial and middle cuneiforms. There was no crepitus or bony step off on palpation. There was no gross instability noted on attempted motion of the first and second tarsometatarsal (TMT) joints; however, motion at the first and second TMT joints elicited pain. She had full active range of motion of the ankle, subtalar joint, and the toes with full motor strength throughout the right foot and ankle. Her sensation to light touch was preserved in all nerve distributions; however, she reported some mild diminishment overlying the area of dorsal midfoot swelling. She had good distal pulses and brisk capillary refill.

Diagnostic Evaluations

Initial nonweight-bearing x-rays of the right foot revealed no concerning abnormalities including no evidence of fracture, dislocation, or subluxation. Weight-bearing x-rays of the right foot revealed slight widening between the bases of the first and second metatarsals and the second metatarsal (see Figures 8.2 and 8.3) and medial cuneiform with a small avulsion fracture of the superolateral aspect of the medial cuneiform. MRI of the right foot revealed diastasis of the medial cuneiform and second metatarsal base with disruption of the interosseous and dorsal components of the Lisfranc ligament. No frank dislocation of the TMT articulations was present. In addition, a bone contusion within the navicular was noted.

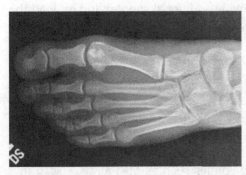 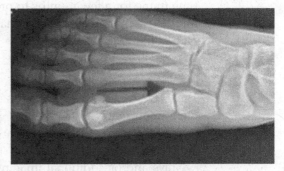

FIGURES 8.2 and 8.3 Nonweight-bearing radiograph that does not demonstrate the Lisfranc injury, side by side with weight-bearing film that does demonstrate the injury in the same patient.

Diagnosis

Lisfranc fracture dislocation, right foot.

CLINICAL PEARL

All unstable Lisfranc injuries should be managed surgically as this area of the foot is susceptible to posttraumatic arthritis and adverse functional outcomes with nonanatomic alignment of the midfoot TMT joints (Watson, Shurnas, & Denker, 2010). Ideally, these injuries are best managed within the first few weeks following onset; however, surgical intervention must be delayed until resolution of swelling, which is typical with these injuries.

Interventions

The patient was placed into a posterior splint, and given crutches. She was instructed to be nonweight bearing, and she was provided with a referral to an orthopedic surgeon within 5 days. The patient elected to proceed with operative intervention. The risks and benefits of open reduction and internal fixation (ORIF) with possible midfoot fusion of her right foot Lisfranc fracture-dislocation were discussed. In the preoperative period, she was advised to remain nonweight bearing on the right lower extremity and was provided with a controlled ankle movement (CAM) walker boot as well as a knee scooter.

Patient Education

If a nonoperative treatment course is pursued, patients should be advised that it takes approximately 4 months for a Lisfranc injury to heal nonsurgically and that during this time frame they will be nonweight bearing on the extremity. Typically, a walking boot or a rocker sole shoe is used after this time frame for a few months to provide additional support and off load the midfoot. Additionally, patients may be referred to physical therapy to work on gait training and balance.

CLINICAL PEARL

It is important to note that her injury was missed at initial presentation to an urgent care center with nonweight-bearing x-rays. A high suspicion for this injury should prompt the clinician to obtain weight-bearing x-rays and/or additional imaging studies such as MRI and CT scan in order to rule out or fully elucidate the nature of this injury.

Follow-Up Evaluation

Approximately 4 months after her procedure, her hardware (two screws) was removed in the operating room. Her Lisfranc joint remained well reduced on x-ray and after 3 to 4 weeks of nonweight bearing, the patient was finally transitioned to weight bearing as tolerated on the right lower extremity. She was referred to physical therapy and remained asymptomatic.

REFERENCES

Seybold, J., & Coetzee, J. (2015). Lisfranc injuries: When to observe, fix, or fuse. *Clinics in Sports Medicine, 34*(4), 705–709.

Watson, T. S., Shurnas, P. S., & Denker, J. (2010). Treatment of Lisfranc joint injury: Current concepts. *Journal of the American Academy of Orthopaedic Surgeons, 18,* 718–728.

Case Study 8.3: Jones Fracture

Vinayak M. Sathe, Teja Karukonda, and Daniel Witmer

SETTING: URGENT CARE

Definition and Incidence

Typically, patients will report a mechanism of injury consisting of either a fall or inversion type injury of the involved foot with subsequent pain localized over the lateral border of the foot and difficulty weight bearing. While there may be swelling and ecchymosis over the area, patients could also present with very little in the way of visible abnormality or deformity. Pain with resisted eversion may also be found on physical exam (Carr, Grieve, & Greaves, 2010). It is important to review the definition of a classic"Jones"fracture as this term does not apply to all fractures involving the base of the fifth metatarsal. Jones fractures constitute transverse or oblique fractures at the junction of the metaphysis and diaphysis of the fifth metatarsal without extension distal to the fourth and fifth intermetatarsal articulation (Carr et al., 2010). Fractures involving the proximal fifth metatarsal proximal to the intermetatarsal articulation are typically characterized as"tuberosity avulsion fractures."Fractures of the proximal fifth metatarsal distal to the intermetatarsal articulation may be characterized as "proximal diaphyseal stress fractures"if prodromal symptoms are present (true Jones fractures are acute injuries without a history of prodromal symptoms).

Patient

A 72-year-old female presented in the outpatient clinic with several weeks of worsening right foot pain. She reported a minor fall from standing with inversion of the right ankle 2 weeks prior. Since then, she has experienced steadily increasing pain along the lateral aspect of the right foot. The pain is exacerbated with weight bearing; however, she is able to ambulate on the right foot without the assistance of a cane or walker. She has not noticed any significant swelling, ecchymosis, or erythema or any wounds overlying the area. She denied any fevers, chills, numbness, tingling, or other musculo-skeletal pain including ankle pain. The pain has responded to rest and ice as well as nonsteroidal anti-inflammatory drugs (NSAIDs) and Tylenol; however, it recurs. Her past medical history is significant for insulin-dependent diabetes mellitus, which is well controlled, and she has regular follow-up visits with her primary care physician. The patient reports that this pain has started to significantly impact her activities of daily living.

Social History

The patient is a retired kindergarten teacher. She lives at home with her husband and a dog. She does not have family nearby.

Physical Assessment

She is in no acute distress, and is morbidly obese. Focused assessment of her right foot reveals no obvious abnormality or deformity. She has normal alignment with no evidence of varus or valgus deformity. Her skin is intact with no abrasions, lacerations, erythema, or ecchymosis. She has an antalgic gait favoring her left lower extremity over her right and she is able to ambulate independently without an assistive device. With palpation, she reports significant tenderness at the base of the fifth metatarsal. There is no bony step-off or crepitus appreciated. The patient denies any other tenderness to palpation in her forefoot, midfoot, hindfoot, or ankle. She has full active range of motion and motor strength of the right foot and ankle; however, the patient does report pain along the lateral aspect of her foot with resisted foot eversion. Her sensation is intact to light touch, and she has intact posterior tibial and dorsalis pedis pulses with her foot warm and well perfused with brisk capillary refill.

Diagnostic Evaluations

Radiographs are taken of the right foot, anterior–posterior (AP), lateral, and oblique views. These reveal a nondisplaced fracture of the base of the fifth metatarsal. The fracture was transverse and localized near the articulation of the fourth and fifth metatarsals.

Diagnosis

Jones fracture.

Interventions

The risks and benefits of nonsurgical and surgical management were discussed with the patient and she initially elected to pursue nonoperative treatment. As such, she was placed into a short leg cast, given crutches, and was advised to remain nonweight bearing on the right lower extremity.

Patient Education

Educate the patient regarding the treatment options, and the typical outcomes of the routes that may be chosen. One of the major concerns regarding treatment of Jones fractures is the high risk for nonunion inherent to these injuries. The portion of the proximal fifth metatarsal, which separates these two blood supplies, is known as the watershed area and is a relatively avascular zone and the site where Jones fractures occur (Rosenberg & Sferra, 2000).

Follow-Up Evaluation

She followed up regularly every 2 to 3 weeks for reevaluation and repeat x-rays. Eventually she was transitioned into a CAM walker boot approximately 6 to 8 weeks status postinjury, as there was evidence of union on x-rays. If the patient went on to nonunion, or continued pain, operative management would be indicated.

CLINICAL PEARL

The diagnosis may be confirmed with plain film x-rays in the form of AP, lateral, and oblique views. CT, MRI, and other imaging modalities are not typically indicated for the initial diagnosis of this injury.

REFERENCES

Carr, G., Grieve, A., & Greaves, I. (2010). The Jones fracture of the fifth metatarsal: Robert Jones. *Trauma, 12*(1), 51–54.

Rosenberg, G. A., & Sferra, J. J. (2000). Treatment strategies for acute fractures and nonunions of the proximal fifth metatarsal. *Journal of the American Academy of Orthopaedic Surgeons, 8*, 332–338.

Case Study 8.4: Sever's Disease

Phoebe M. Heffron

SETTING: ORTHOPEDIC URGENT CARE

Definition and Incidence

Sever's disease is the term for calcaneal apophysitis or traction overuse on the growth plate of the calcaneus. Also known as "calcaneal apophysitis," this is a common, self-limited overuse condition characterized by heel pain. The pain is caused by inflammation of the growth plate at the back of the heel. This is a pediatric problem typically affecting both boys and girls, frequently during their pubertal growth spurts. Boys are affected two to three times as frequently as girls (Sitati & Kingori, 2009).

Patient

This is a 14-year-old male who presents to his pediatric primary care office complaining of heel pain that began several weeks ago. He says, "I just finished my football season and really didn't want to miss any playing time. My heels have been bothering me for a while. The pain is pretty bad and gets worse when I run for a long time. Sometimes it hurts so much that I feel like I have to walk on my tiptoes to avoid putting pressure on them. Usually if we have a long weekend off, I get a little relief." His mother adds, "I vaguely remember a similar issue when I was younger so we have tried icing when he has pain and he has taken ibuprofen a few times. I tried to encourage him to take some time off from football but he was too stubborn to agree."

Social History

The patient is an honors student and was the only freshman to make his school's varsity football team. He was really worried about losing his spot on the team and letting his teammates down. "I just played through the pain."

CLINICAL PEARL

Sever's disease ceases in adolescence when the growth plate in the calcaneus fuses.

Physical Assessment

The lower extremities show no evidence of acute abnormality. There is no swelling or ecchymosis. The temperature of the feet is normal, posterior tibial pulses are normal, and capillary refill is less than 3 seconds bilaterally. There is no point tenderness over the calcaneus or the malleolus. There is pain with squeezing of the bilateral heels. The patient walks with a limp, slightly up on his toes. Range of motion is normal aside from slightly decreased dorsiflexion.

Diagnostic Evaluations

X-rays are typically done though there is some controversy over the necessity of imaging as diagnosis is typically made clinically. For example, in a small retrospective study, 5.1% of x-rays showed an acute abnormality, prompting the authors to advise that imaging is important so that more severe injuries are not missed (Rachel, Williams, Sawyer, Warner, & Kelly, 2011). Figure 8.4 demonstrates some widening of the calcaneal apophysis.

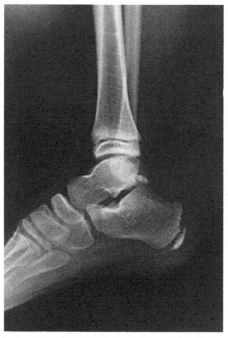

FIGURE 8.4 Lateral radiograph demonstrating the skeletally immature apophysis of the calcaneous.

Diagnosis

Sever's disease.

Interventions

The nurse practitioner advises the patient to obtain orthotics (custom made or over the counter) to wear daily in supportive shoes, prescribes a stretching regimen, and recommends icing before and after activity. The nurse practitioner further restricts the patient from participating in athletics until the pain has resolved. The patient also receives a referral to orthopedics to schedule an appointment if the pain has not improved in 3 weeks of this conservative treatment.

Patient Education

As a nurse practitioner, it is important to educate the patient and his parents that this condition is self-limited. It is also crucial to discuss the restrictions on athletics until the pain has resolved as well as the possibility that the patient could require an immobilizing boot if heel lifts, activity restriction, stretching, and anti-inflammatory medications do not relieve the pain. It is also important to note that while the growth plate is open, the pain can return.

Follow-Up Evaluation

The nurse practitioner will likely see this patient again—either in a follow-up for this complaint or in the near future for a routine well-child visit or other acute visit. The nurse practitioner can permit him to return to athletics gradually once his pain has resolved. It is important for the nurse practitioner to be familiar with this condition as it is quite common in the pediatric setting.

REFERENCES

Rachel, J. N., Williams, J. B., Sawyer, J. R., Warner, W. C., & Kelly, D. M. (2011). Is radiographic evaluation necessary in children with a clinical diagnosis of calcaneal apophosytosis (Sever's disease)? *Journal of Pediatric Orthopedics, 31*(5), 50. doi:10.1097/BPO.0b013e318219905c

Sitati, F. S., & Kingori, J. (2009). Chronic bilateral heel pain in a child with Sever's disease: A case report and review of the literature. *Cases Journal, 2*, 9365. doi:10.1186/1757-1626-2-9365

Case Study 8.5: Sesamoiditis

Kaitlin M. Ford

SETTING: PRIMARY CARE

Definition and Incidence

Sesamoiditis is a generalized term to describe painful inflammation of the tendons and soft tissue surrounding the two sesamoid bones of the hallux in the absence of radiographic changes (Boike, Schnirring-Judge, & McMillin, 2011). Sesamoiditis is typically caused by repetitive stress to the first metatarsal region. The two hallux sesamoid bones are located within the flexor hallucis brevis on the plantar surface of the first metatarsal head and anchored in position by both medial and lateral sesamoidal ligaments as well as small portions of the abductor and adductor hallucis tendons (Cohen, 2009). As an important component of the first metatarsophalangeal joint (MTPJ), they absorb and help distribute forces of weight-bearing exercises on the great toe (Boike et al., 2011). Sesamoiditis most commonly affects active teens and young adults, making up 9% of foot and ankle injuries (Boike et al., 2011).

Patient

Patient is a 16-year-old male who presents with the chief concern of right "foot pain." He plays basketball for his high school team and states that he has noticed increasing pain located at the base of his right big toe during practice. He describes the pain as originally starting 2.5 months ago as a dull ache only after practices but has progressively gotten worse. It is now a sharp pain being a constant 3 out of 10 that can be as high as 7 out of 10 during practice and with any weight-bearing movements. He says it feels as if he is "walking with a sharp stone in his shoe." The pain does not spread or radiate to any other parts of his foot or leg. He has never had pain similar to this before and denies any pain in his left foot. He cannot recall any specific incident that caused the pain, has not recently changed his basketball sneakers, and denies any trauma. He tried ibuprofen, 800 mg as needed, and has been icing his foot after every practice for 10 minutes as instructed by the school physical trainer to find mild if any relief.

Social History

The 16-year-old male is in his junior year of high school. He recently joined a traveling basketball club 4 months ago and states that he has been practicing more often as he has practice or games almost everyday for his high school or club team. He has been trying to play through the pain as his high school team is currently in the playoffs; however, his pain has gotten so bad that he has started to sit out during practices. He describes extreme frustration with his current state of play and is concerned that he will lose his starting position if he keeps sitting out during practice.

Physical Assessment

The patient is a 16-year-old male in no acute distress, but demonstrates some discomfort throughout the physical exam. He is 5'10" and weighs 160 lb. On inspection, there was slight inflammation but no erythema, abrasions, or bruising on the plantar surface of the right metatarsal. On physical exam, he has significant pain at the base of the plantar surface of his right great toe that is exacerbated by resisted plantar flexion and extreme passive dorsiflexion of the great toe. Range of motion and strength of the ankle and big toe are normal; however, the patient admits to some "stiffness" on dorsiflexion of the great toe. On gait assessment, he has an antalgic gait with pain at the base of the right great toe that worsens with medial foot walking, single-leg heel raise on his right, and standing. Tenderness to palpation is elicited only at the base of the MTPJ. There are no focal neurologic deficits in the right lower extremity.

Diagnostic Evaluations

A radiograph was obtained to exclude other painful sesamoid disorders. No fracture, fragmentation, structural abnormalities, or necrosis was seen.

Diagnosis

Sesamoiditis.

Interventions

The patient was advised to continue his current therapies of icing and taking ibuprofen or other anti-inflammatory over-the-counter medication as needed. It was recommended that he increase the frequency and duration of icing to include icing for 10 to 15 minutes every 2 to 3 hours or after any activity that aggravates the pain. He was also instructed to rest his foot by eliminating all participation in basketball. He was instructed that rest was the best way to reduce repetitive stress on the MTPJ and allow time for healing to occur. He was cautioned that without proper treatment, sesamoiditis could become a chronic problem that requires steroid injections or even surgery. It was additionally recommended that custom-molded orthotics or gel inserts under the sesamoids be worn at all times to alleviate the stress placed on the MTPJ. After discussion of the treatment plan, the patient admitted to resistance in completely stopping all basketball play. He did, however, agree to rest his foot more by wearing orthotics throughout the day and sitting out for practices and playing only during games. The patient was then instructed that should pain worsen or persist for longer than 6 weeks despite following the above therapies, he should follow-up with a podiatrist or orthopedic surgeon who might recommend an intra-articular corticosteroid injection or potentially a sesamoidectomy.

Patient Education

Educate the patient on the treatment options that includes nonsurgical conservative treatment is recommended as first line management for new onset sesamoiditis as success rates are very high (Boike et al., 2011). If detected early and managed properly, sesamoiditis is usually curable within 4 to 6 months (Pontell, 2006). Intra-articular corticosteroids may provide relief for acute pain and inflammation; however, repeated injections are not recommended for chronic management (Cohen, 2009). Sesamoidectomy is typically reserved for chronic sesamoiditis, but pain may not completely resolve even after surgery (Boike et al., 2011).

Follow-Up Evaluation

A follow-up visit was scheduled for 6 weeks. At that time, the patient reported feeling relief of his discomfort and was returned slowly to activities.

REFERENCES

Boike, A., Schnirring-Judge, M., & McMillin, S. (2011). Sesamoid disorders of the first metatarsophalangeal joint. *Clinics in Podiatric Medicine and Surgery, 28*, 269–285.

Cohen, B. E. (2009). Hallux sesamoid disorders. *Foot and Ankle Clinics, 14*(1), 91–104.

Pontell, D., Hallivis, R., & Dollard, M. D. (2006). Sports injuries in the pediatric and adolescent foot and ankle: Common overuse and acute presentations. *Clinics in Podiatric Medicine and Surgery, 23*(1), 209–231.

Case Study 8.6: Plantar Fasciitis

Karen M. Pawelek

SETTING: PRIMARY CARE

Definition and Incidence

Plantar fasciitis is a common cause of foot pain and is defined as pain in the plantar region of the foot along the medial aspect of the calcaneus that worsens with walking (Jariwala, Bruce, & Jain, 2011). While plantar fasciitis is not well understood, it can be related to chronic degeneration of the plantar fascia due to overuse or limited dorsiflexion (Douglas, 2003). Approximately 2 million office visits annually occur due to plantar fasciitis (Riddle, Pulisic, Pidcoe, & Johnson, 2003). The peak incidence of plantar fasciitis is between ages 40 and 60 years and is often caused from overuse or shoes with a poor arch (Riddle et al., 2003).

Patient

The patient presents with right heel pain. Initially, she noticed the pain in her right heel that started 3 weeks ago after she began increasing her marathon training schedule. The pain is worse with dorsiflexion of the right foot and also with palpation along the heel to the forefoot. She describes the pain as a 9 out of 10 when present. The pain is worse first thing in the morning when she takes her first steps or after she has been resting and then begins walking again. She has never had this pain before. The patient tried ibuprofen 400 mg twice every few days and had some relief, but it does not last. She started wearing new running shoes just before starting her training routine. During her teaching day, she wears high-heel shoes.

Social History

She works as a teacher. She is married and lives with her husband and 15-year-old son. She has never smoked and she drinks one to two glasses of wine per day.

Physical Assessment

This 45-year-old female presents and is in no acute distress. Discomfort is noted with palpation at the insertion of the plantar fascia on the right foot with deep pressure. She does have some pain in same area with extension

.of the great toe along the plantar fascia (stretch test). With range of motion testing, she exhibits mild tightness of the Achilles tendon with dorsiflexion. Pes planus (flattening of the medial arch) is noted on the right foot.

Diagnostic Evaluations

Lateral and axis views of foot ruled out calcaneus stress fracture and spur.

Diagnosis

Plantar fasciitis of the right foot.

Interventions

Ice massage and NSAIDs for inflammation and pain control were recommended initially. Ibuprofen of 800 mg with food three times a day was recommended. The patient was instructed to avoid high-impact activities until the pain subsided, then gradually resume usual activities. Achilles tendon stretching exercises were advised. Silicone heel inserts and avoidance of flat shoes were also recommended.

Patient Education

Educate your patient that a trial of NSAIDs is recommended. It is also important to teach the patient that weight reduction is beneficial in plantar fasciitis treatment and prevention. Importantly, both active and passive stretching exercises of the Achilles tendon should be performed, and return to activity is recommended to be slow and progressive (Healey & Chen, 2010). Supportive footwear with a cushioned heel is important for comfort and care. Referral to orthopedics may be an option if the symptoms are not improved with conservative measures.

Follow-Up Evaluation

The patient returned at the 8-week mark and reported that her pain gradually resolved. She continued to use NSAIDs as needed, and to do stretching exercises; she was encouraged to continue this treatment routine.

REFERENCES

Douglas, R. (2003). Fasciitis: Treatment pearls. Retrieved from http://www.aapsm.org/plantar_fasciitis.html

Healey, K., & Chen, K. (2010). Plantar fasciitis: Current diagnostic modalities and treatments. *Clinics in Podiatric Medicine and Surgery, 27*(3), 369–380.

Jariwala, A., Bruce, D., & Jain, A. (2011). A guide to recognition and treatment of plantar fasciitis. *Primary Care, 21*(7), 22–24.

Riddle, D. L., Pulisic, M., Pidcoe, P., & Johnson, R. E. (2003). Risk factors for plantar fasciitis: A matched case control study. *Journal of Bone and Joint Surgery, 85-A*(5), 872–877.

SECTION III

Spine Cases

CHAPTER 9

SPINE

Case Study 9.1: Acute Compression Fracture

Jason N. DaCruz

SETTING: ACUTE OR URGENT CARE

Definition and Incidence

A compression fracture is a fracture in the spine that is usually caused by osteoporosis. Compression fractures occur at a rate of 117 per 100,000 people (Savage, 2014).

Patient

Patient presents with the chief complaint of "low back pain." She describes a sudden onset of severe back pain that began 4 days ago while grocery shopping. In the midst of bending down to pick up some groceries, she had a severe bout of intense pain, which she rated as 10 out of 10, and it was associated with significant spasm. She has had severe difficulty mobilizing since. Pain is noted with all activity, even while in bed, and exacerbated with rolling over. She was initially seen at her primary care provider's office and was diagnosed with lumbar strain. Her initial treatment plan was pharmacologic, treated with Naprosyn (nonsteroidal anti-inflammatory) and Flexeril (muscle relaxer); the patient reports no relief from either. She denies any leg pain, paraethesias, or urinary or bowel difficulties. She has had difficulties moving about in bed and mobilizing to the extent that she is unable to perform her daily living activities.

Social History

She is currently retired.

Physical Assessment

On physical examination, the patient is a 73-year-old woman who is alert, awake, and orientated, in moderate distress secondary to pain. She is 5'3", weighs 230 lb, and stands with a slight forward flexed posture. There is tenderness noted at the thoracolumbar junction; no palpable step off or *gibbus* (Latin for "hump"); no skin changes or ecchymosis surrounding the thoracolumbar spine. No paravertebral spasm is appreciated. Her lumbar mechanics are poor in flexion to 40 degrees; she is able to move with minimal extension, which causes increasing pain. Otherwise, she has a negative straight leg raise, trace reflexes at the knees and ankles bilaterally and symmetrical. She has no clonus and is neurovascularly intact.

Diagnostic Evaluations

Radiographs were obtained in anterior–posterior (AP) and lateral lumbar spine, which demonstrate a compression fracture at L1 (see Figure 9.1).

Diagnosis

L1 compression fracture, with minimal segmental kyphosis.

CLINICAL PEARL

If you are contemplating whether or not a fracture seen on plain radiographs is acute or chronic, consider obtaining MRI to check for acute signal changes seen on T1 and T2 images (Kim & Vaccaro, 2006). If there are acute signal changes, this will help to diagnose the issue as one that is acute in nature, versus chronic.

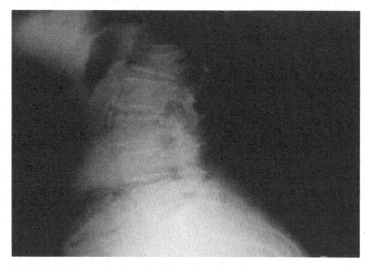

FIGURE 9.1 Lateral radiograph of the lumbar spine demonstrating a compression fracture.

Interventions

Once you have made the diagnosis of acute lumbar compression fracture, consider using a support brace such as Aspen corset to treat your patient. If you observe that the patient's kyphosis is significant, greater than 25 degrees, consider Jewitt versus thoracolumbar sacral orthosis (TLSO) brace. TLSO brace is commonly used if multiple compression fractures or burst fracture are identified. It is also used in the cases in which you want to control rotation. The Jewitt brace is used mainly for simple compression fractures surrounding the thoracolumbar junction (T11, T12, L1, L2). It does not control rotation but does provide hyperextension, which is beneficial at the junction when normally these types of fractures cause kyphosis. In this case, the patient was treated with a lumbar corset with the rationale that her segmental kyphosis was 18 degrees at the time of visit, and she had been previously mobilizing without any further changes, appearing structurally stable. Discussion with the patient included repeat radiographs in 4 weeks as well as instructions to contact the office earlier if pain worsened, potentially suggestive of further compression collapse. An example of an Aspen corset is found in Figure 9.2.

Patient Education

It would be helpful to explain the potential use of a kyphoplasty procedure if the patient's pain does not improve over the next 2 to 3 weeks. Kyphoplasty is a minimally invasive procedure where cement polymethylmethacrylate (PMMA) is placed into the vertebral body within a balloon by means of a small incision (Savage, Schroeder, & Anderson, 2014). Advancement of a small tube through the pedicle is performed under fluoroscopy and then the PMMA is introduced into the fracture for stabilization. Advise the patient to avoid repetitive forward bending, avoid lifting more than 10 lb, and maintain upright posture until return to clinic for a follow-up visit in 4 weeks. The patient was also instructed to contact the office earlier should the pain worsen or symptoms change.

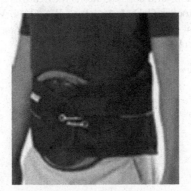

FIGURE 9.2 An Aspen corset.

Follow-Up Evaluation

For this patient, her 4-week check revealed that she had overall improvement in her pain by 50%. She reported residual pain upon turning in bed but is able to sleep comfortably on her recliner. She is ambulating without significant pain. She will continue restrictions of no repetitive bending, no forward flexion, no lifting of more than 10 lb, and continued use of lumbar corset brace for support.

At the follow-up visit, a repeat x-ray of the lateral lumbar spine was obtained. The patient showed no worsening of compression or segmental kyphosis.

Longer term follow-up will consist of advising the patient to: schedule follow-up visits every 4 weeks for 3 months; continue the limitations in activity and movement until the pain resolves; and report persistent or intensified pain. If pain persists or intensifies, consult with interventional radiologist for kyphoplasty. Generally, compression fractures are monitored over 3 months with repeat x-rays. No physical therapy is recommended.

CLINICAL PEARL

The typical presentation of compression fracture is elderly patients with a known history of osteopenia or osteoporosis. A common rule of thumb is that once the pain has dissipated, the compression fracture has healed. If pain persists or intensifies, consultation with a spine surgeon is recommended at a point postinjury that seems appropriate, based upon the patient presentation and your experience.

REFERENCES

Kim, D. H., & Vaccaro, A. R. (2006). Osteoporotic compression fractures of the spine: Current options and considerations for treatment. *Spine Journal, 6*, 479–487.

Savage, J. W., Schroeder, G. D., & Anderson, P. A. (2014). Vertebroplasty and kyphoplasty for the treatment of osteoporotic vertebra. *Journal of the American Academy of Orthopaedic Surgeons, 22*, 653–664.

Case Study 9.2: Acute Disc Herniation

Jason N. DaCruz

SETTING: URGENT CARE/PRIMARY CARE

Definition and Incidence

A lumbar disc herniation is a common low back disorder and defined by the disc (nucleous pulposa) being extruded into the spinal canal.

Patient

A 37-year-old male patient presents with a 3-week history of progressively worsening subjective left-sided low back pain as well as left leg pain, which he described as a consistent 8 out of 10 pain. He describes no particular injury or event that exacerbated his condition. He has a history of relatively mild low back complaints for years prior to this flare up. He describes the pain worsening with bending forward as well as prolonged periods of sitting. The leg pain travels in a distribution of posterior buttock, thigh, and lateral calf, and at times has a sensation of tingling into the great toe. He has been seen by a chiropractor over the past 3 weeks with no benefit. Ibuprofen and some Flexeril have been of no great benefit to him.

Social History

He is a police officer in a town near his home. He is married and has two daughters, ages 8 and 6.

Physical Assessment

On exam, he's a heavyset gentleman, alert, awake, and orientated. He is 6' tall and 275 lb. His lumbar mechanics are restricted and elicit pain. He demonstrates constraint in forward flexion to 40 degrees, and greater with reproducible left leg pain. There are no significant difficulties with lumbar extension. A positive straight leg raise is demonstrated at 60 degrees. Deep tendon reflexes are symmetrical and 1+ at the knees and ankles. With strength testing, he has 4 out of 5 dorsiflexion. Foot weakness is appreciated on the left. There is no weakness exhibited with plantar flexion, and he has 5 out of 5 quadriceps strength. Hip mechanics are unremarkable in internal and external rotation, which are full and pain-free motion. He denies any bowel or bladder dysfunction.

CLINICAL PEARL

It is important that you rule out Cauda Equina syndrome. This is a rare condition that occurs with approximately 2% of all herniated discs (Greenhalgh, Truman, Webster, & Selfe, 2015). The condition is considered a medical emergency, and is evidenced by bowel and/or bladder dysfunction, reduced sensation in the saddle area, or sexual dysfunction (Fraser, Roberts, & Murphy, 2009).

Diagnostic Evaluations

Radiographs are obtained and include both AP and LAT views, which reveal relative disc space collapse at L4-5 and L5-S1, with no sign of any instability or spondylolisthesis (see Figures 9.3 and 9.4).

Diagnosis

Acute disc herniation at L5.

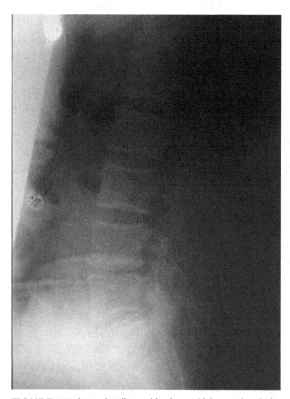

FIGURE 9.3 Lateral radiographic view, which reveals relative disc space collapse at L4–5 and L5–S1, no sign of any instability or spondylolisthesis.

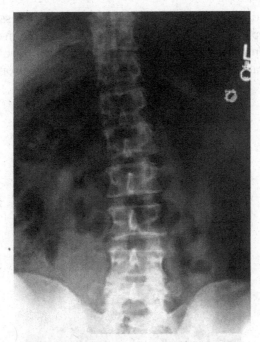

FIGURE 9.4 Anteroposterior radiograph, revealing the relative disc space collapse at L4–5 and L5–S1, no sign of any instability or other degenerative changes.

Interventions

He was placed on a tapering dose of dexamethasone 2 mg over the ensuing 8 days (two tablets four times a day for 2 days, one tablet four times a day for 2 days, one tablet twice a day for 2 days, one tablet once a day for 2 days), as well as Baclofen 10 mg every 8 hours as needed for spasm. He was also placed into an Aspen brace corset for comfort (see Figure 9.2). Because of the objective findings of dorsiflexion weakness, associated with an L5 root dysfunction, an MRI was subsequently obtained.

Patient Education

Educate your patient on treatment options for disc herniation. Options to further consider would be a possible L4-5 epidural cortisone injection. Commonly when patients have intractable type pain it is difficult to have them entertain physical therapy, secondary to a pure pain issue. Often, an epidural injection will decrease the amount of radicular pain, so that the patient can then be mobilized. With less discomfort, physical therapy would be a good initial treatment plan, working two to three times a week for a minimum of 6 weeks with a physical therapist.

Follow-Up Evaluation

The patient returned after obtaining an MRI within 3 days. The MRI confirmed the suspected L5 disc herniation (see Figures 9.5 and 9.6). After reviewing the MRI findings with the patient and given the patient's continued pain complex with associated weakness, he was referred to an orthopedic spine surgeon for further management. He subsequently underwent an L4-5 discectomy with complete resolution of his leg pain postoperatively, and improvement of his dorsiflexion strength.

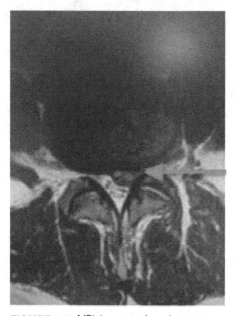

FIGURE 9.5 MRI demonstrating a large left-sided L4–5 disc herniation.

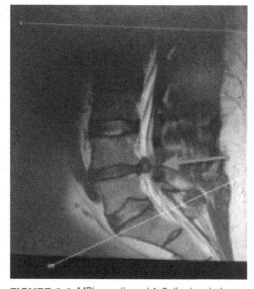

FIGURE 9.6 MRI revealing a L4–5 disc herniation.

REFERENCES

Fraser, S., Roberts, L., & Murphy, E. (2009). Cauda equina syndrome: A literature review of its definition and clinical presentation. *Archives of Physical Medicine & Rehabilitation, 90*(11), 1964–1968. doi:10.1016/j.apmr.2009.03.021

Greenhalgh, S., Truman, C., Webster, V., & Selfe, J. (2015). An investigation into the patient experience of cauda equina syndrome: A qualitative study. *Physiotherapy Practice & Research, 36*(1), 23–31. doi:10.3233/PPR-140047

Case Study 9.3: Spondylolysis

Jason N. DaCruz

SETTING: ACUTE OR URGENT CARE

Definition and Incidence

Spondylolysis is defined as a unilateral or bilateral defect along the pars inter-articularis, and spondylolisthesis is the actual displacement of a vertebral body in correlation to the underlying vertebra (Metzger & Chaney, 2014).

Patient

Chief complaint is "low back pain." Patient is a pleasant 26-year-old female, who recently experienced a slip and a fall while at home 5 days ago. She had a significant sudden onset of low back pain, and was initially seen at a walk-in clinic. She was prescribed nonsteroidal anti-inflammatory drugs (NSAIDs) and a muscle relaxant, diagnosed with low back strain. She has continued all of her activities with difficulty, especially with extension of the back. Symptoms are slightly improved with trunk flexion or her legs raised, and she denies radiating leg pain. Pain is rated at a 9 out of 10. Upon further questioning, she admits to low back discomfort for quite some time but never to this extent.

Social History

This 26-year-old is a very active individual who exercises four to five times a week. She works as an assistant in a law firm and is single without any children.

Physical Assessment

On physical assessment she is 5'5" tall and weighs 135 lb. She stands with a slight forward flexed posture of approximately 10 degrees. A non-tender lumbar spine is noted. Slight discomfort is noted with palpation of paravertebrals. No skin changes are visualized. Lumbar mechanics are slow but able to surpass 60 degrees; returning upright increases pain as well as any extended posture. Bilateral negative straight leg raise test is observed, although at maximum hip flexion, tension is noted in lower back as well as very tight hamstrings bilaterally. Symmetrical reflexes are 2+ for knees and ankles. Good hip flexion is noted bilaterally with some subjective improvement in low back pain. Hips mechanics are otherwise unremarkable with full range of motion, and she is neurovascularly intact.

Diagnostic Evaluations

Radiographs were obtained in AP view, and lateral flexion and extension views were obtained, along with oblique views of lumbar spine. The x-rays reveal isthmic spondylolisthesis on the lateral view (Figure 9.7). In the lateral view in flexion, a spondylolisthesis of L4 on L5 is revealed (Figure 9.8). Figure 9.9, the oblique view of the lumbar spine, demonstrates a positive "Scotty dog sign." The neck of the Scotty dog shows a fracture at that collar.

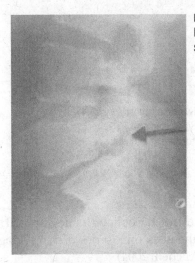

FIGURE 9.7 Lateral view of the lumbar spine demonstrating isthmic spondylolisthesis.

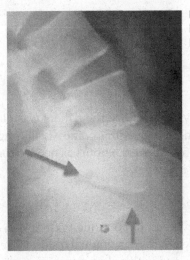

FIGURE 9.8 Flexion view of the lumbar spine demonstrating a spondylolisthesis of L4 on L5.

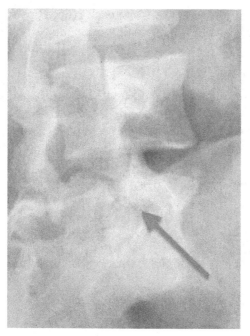

FIGURE 9.9 Oblique view of the lumbar spine demonstrating a positive "Scotty dog sign." The neck of the Scotty dog shows a fracture at that collar.

CLINICAL PEARL

The Scotty dog sign is found on the oblique radiographs. The sign is demonstrated as a break in the neck on a series of Scotty dogs stacked in a column (McTimoney & Micheli, 2004).

Diagnosis

Spondylolysis.

Interventions

With consideration to the acuity of the injury, the patient was placed initially into an aspen brace corset, continued on with Lodine XL 400-mg twice a day as needed for pain, and Soma 350 mg every 6 hours as needed for spasm. She was scheduled for reevaluation in 2 weeks.

Patient Education

Educate your patients that they need to continue with flexion-based exercises, and to return to exercise regimens in a gradual fashion. The importance of keeping up with the exercises and with a slow return to sports needs to be emphasized for best patient outcomes.

Follow-Up Evaluation

At the 2-week visit, symptoms had subsided. Physical therapy was started with a flexion-based exercise program and a focus on piriformis and hamstring mobilization, as well as core strengthening, for 6 weeks. She was then reevaluated at that point. At the 6-week mark, there was noted improvement in her function as well as activity level. She continued to describe that some symptoms still remained. This patient will be clinically monitored for a period of 6 months with the hope that she will be able to return back to a good active lifestyle and return to her baseline function. If symptoms persist, quality of life changes, or pain worsens she will be referred to an orthopedic spine surgeon.

CLINICAL PEARL

Not all young back-pain patients have lumbar strain. Depending on the underlying diagnosis, a typical PT routine may exacerbate a patient's course. In this situation, had the patient been referred to PT without the underlying diagnosis, she in all likelihood would have been placed into an extension/Mckeinze program, which would have made her condition worsen in regards to her pain.

REFERENCES

McTimoney, C., & Micheli, L. (2004). Managing back pain in young athletes. *Journal of Musculoskeletal Medicine, 21*(2), 63–69.

Metzger, R., & Chaney, S. (2014). Spondylolysis and spondylolisthesis: What the primary care provider should know. *Journal of the American Association of Nurse Practitioners, 26*(1), 5–12. doi:10.1002/2327-6924.12083

Case Study 9.4: Chronic Sacroiliac Pain

Jason N. DaCruz

SETTING: ACUTE OR URGENT CARE

Definition and Incidence

Sacroilitis is pain in the sacroiliac joint or joints. Sacroiliac pain may be the source of low back pain in as many as 20% of cases (Bashir, 2011).

Patient

A 34-year-old female presents with ongoing left buttock pain that has been persistent for months. She at times has referable pain to posterior thigh, but this is not as consistent as the buttock pain. She does report a history of having undergone a L5-S1 anterior posterior fusion 2 years ago, from which she did well. The present pain seems to worsen when getting out of bed, climbing up and down stairs, as well as getting up from a seated position. It has affected her job to the point where she has had to call out of work because of pain. It does seem to improve at times with walking, but does not resolve it. She has no associated numbness, tingling, or bowel difficulties. She did try a few sessions of chiropractic care, which gave her some relief, but it was short lived. At times, over-the-counter medication has provided her with some relief.

Social History

The patient is a 34-year-old waitress at a local family-owned restaurant. She has two children, a 1-year-old and a 5-year-old. She is married and lives with her family.

Physical Assessment

Patient stands in an upright posture; she is nontender across the spinous processes of the lumbar spine, quite notably tender across the sacroiliac joint on the left. Lumbar mechanics are synchronous in forward flexion and extension. She reports some increased tension surpassing 60 degrees of flexion in the left buttock. Hip mechanics bilaterally are without restrictions or reproducible groin pain; there is some lateralized hip and buttock pain with external rotation on the left. A positive FABRE test (Figure 9.10) is noted on the left. She has a negative straight leg raise test bilaterally and symmetrical reflexes of 1+ elicited at the knees and ankles. There is good motor tone; 5 out of 5 in the quadriceps and plantar-dorsiflexion in the feet. Symmetrical sensation to light touch is demonstrated in the first web space and lateral foot bilaterally (Figure 9.11).

Diagnostic Evaluations

Plain films, MRI, and CT scans are typically used to rule out discogenic pain as the primary source of the pain. The diagnosis of sacroiliac dysfunction is based primarily on subjective history, clinical examination, as well as ruling out an underlying degenerative disc problem.

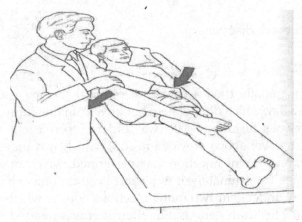

FIGURE 9.10 FABRE test.

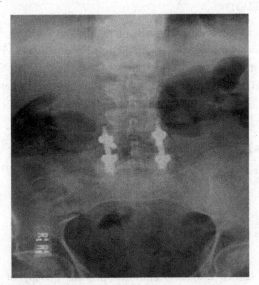

FIGURE 9.11 Postoperative patient with L5-S1 fusion, demonstrating hardware.

CLINICAL PEARL

Patients with true sacroiliac pain are very responsive to a sacroiliac corti-sone injection. This can be used as a therapeutic diagnostic intervention. This is very helpful when you may be trying to differentiate SI joint pain from discogenic pain. It is common to develop SI joint pain mainly in patients who have had a L5-S1 fusion in the past. The fusion mass increases load and forces that normally do not exist across the SI joint in normal biomechanics. The other patient subset that develops SI joint pain is those who have direct trauma/impact to the joint from a fall.

Diagnosis

Chronic sacroiliac pain.

Interventions

Patient initially tried a course of physical therapy and Lodine 400 mg twice a day, which did not help her greatly. In the intrim, given her history of previous fusion, an MRI was ordered to rule out adjacent segment disease (level above previous fusion), which was unremarkable. At that point, an SI joint injection was performed, which dramatically relieved her pain. Unfortunately, it was short lived for only 3 months. She subsequently underwent two more injections both of which relieved her pain, but only for short periods. She thereafter was referred back to her ortho-pedic spine surgeon for consultation on a possible sacroiliac fusion.

Patient Education

The patient was educated about treatment options that included nonop-erative and noninvasive to surgical intervention. A course of physical ther-apy was initially tried and this was followed by an SI injection. Sacroiliac fusion surgery was also described as a possibility for treatment.

Follow-Up Evaluation

Patient is back for a follow-up at the 6-week mark to evaluate the physi-cal therapy and review the MRI. She was then seen at the 3-month time period.

REFERENCE

Bashir, F. (2011). Diagnosis and manipulative therapy of sacroiliac joint disorder. *International Musculoskeletal Medicine, 33*(3), 115–119. doi:10.1179/1753615 11X13153160074937

Case Study 9.5: Chronic Low Back Pain

Karen M. Myrick

SETTING: PRIMARY CARE

Definition and Incidence

Low back pain is a common complaint seen by providers in primary care. Approximately 80% of people in the United States will experience at least one episode of back pain in their lives (Kawi, 2014).

Patient

A 40-year-old male patient presents with a history of low back pain for several years. He comes in today as his discomfort has increased over the last 2 days. He describes the pain as aching in quality and is an 8 out of 10 at the worst, and located across the low back without any radiation. The pain is worse with sitting, and better with standing or lying down. He describes no particular injury or event that exacerbated his condition, and he has had 4- to 6-week-long sessions of physical therapy in the past. He admits to doing his home exercise program for a few weeks after each session, but eventually stops doing his exercises.

Social History

He is a construction worker who is single. He smokes one pack of cigarettes a day, and drinks four to five beers each evening.

Physical Assessment

This 40-year-old male is 5'11" tall and weighs 207 lb. He has a protuberant abdomen, and a hunched posture. With range of motion testing, his lumbar mechanics are restricted in all directions. Flexion and extension, lateral bending and rotation are limited, and any motion elicits pain. He is able to heel and toe walk, and has a negative straight leg raising test. There is no bony tenderness with palpation of the lumbar spine. Deep tendon reflexes are symmetrical and 2+ patellar and Achilles. Hip mechanics are unremarkable in internal and external rotation, which are full and pain-free motion. With strength testing, he has 5 out of 5 strength with quadriceps, hamstring, foot dorsiflexion, and extension testing.

Diagnostic Evaluations

Radiographs are not taken.

Diagnosis

Chronic low back pain.

Interventions

The patient was instructed to begin his home exercise program, and to be consistent with these exercises. A follow-up visit is made for 6 weeks.

Patient Education

Educate your patient on the importance of continuing exercises at home for reduction of symptoms and for prevention of future episodes of pain. It is extremely important to emphasize that physical activity and weight loss are essential for body mechanics and decreasing the strain on the lumbar spine.

Follow-Up Evaluation

At the 6-week follow-up visit, the patient reported some relief of his discomfort. He also stated that he was working with a personal trainer to help with directed exercises for the core. He was encouraged to continue to work on his fitness.

REFERENCE

Kawi, J. (2014). Influence of self-management and self-management support on chronic low back pain patients in primary care. *Journal of the American Association of Nurse Practitioners, 26*(12), 664–673. doi:10.1002/2327-6924.12117

Case Study 9.6: Chronic Degenerative Disc Disease

Karen M. Myrick

SETTING: PRIMARY CARE

Definition and Incidence

A chronic lumbar disc herniation is a common low back disorder and defined by the disc (nucleous pulposa) being extruded into the spinal canal. This can be recurrent in nature. Low back pain has an incidence of 84% of the population (Kovacs, 2014).

Patient

A 68-year-old male patient presents with a several year history of progressively worsening low back pain as well as pain that radiates down the right leg to his foot. He describes the pain as aching in quality and is a 7 out of 10 at the worst. He describes no particular injury or event that exacerbated his condition, and he has been working with his primary care provider and physical therapist on and off for years. Recently, he has not been doing his exercises, and notices that he has put on 10 to 15 lb over the holidays. He has a history of relatively mild low back complaints for years prior to this flare-up. Pain is exacerbated with forward bending and with prolonged periods of sitting, such as long car rides or sitting through a movie. He is getting more frustrated with the discomfort, as he wants to play with grandchildren and the pain is interfering with his activities of daily living.

Social History

He is a retired librarian, who is widowed and has two daughters who live close by with three grandchildren, ages 4, 3, and 1.

Physical Assessment

This 68-year-old male is 6′ tall and 217 lb. He has a slow and steady gait. He is able to heel and toe walk. Range of motion demonstrates that his lumbar mechanics are restricted in flexion and extension, lateral bending and rotation, and elicit pain. A negative straight leg raise is demonstrated. Deep tendon reflexes are symmetrical and 2+ patellar and Achilles.

With strength testing, he has 5 out of 5 strength with quadriceps, hamstring, foot dorsiflexion, and extension testing. Hip mechanics are unremarkable in internal and external rotation, which are full and pain-free motion.

Diagnostic Evaluations

Radiographs are obtained and include both AP and LAT views.

Diagnosis

Degenerative disc disease.

Interventions

The patient was instructed to begin a formalized course of physical therapy, working specifically to increase core stability. A follow-up visit in 6 to 8 weeks is recommended to evaluate the effectiveness of the physical therapy program.

Patient Education

Educate your patient on the importance of physical activity and weight loss, to help with decreasing the strain on the lumbar spine.

Follow-Up Evaluation

The patient returned in 8 weeks. At this visit, he described some relief of his discomfort, but not to 100%. He states that he is better, but he continues to have pain that occasionally awakens him at night, and he is having difficulty getting through the day without discomfort. At this point, he is referred to an orthopedic spine surgeon for further management and discussion of treatment options.

REFERENCE

Kovacs, F., Arana, E., Royuela, A., Estremera, A., Amengual, G., Asenjo, B., . . . Abraira, V. (2014). Disc degeneration and chronic low back pain: An association which becomes nonsignificant when endplate changes and disc contour are taken into account. *Neuroradiology, 56*(1), 25–33. doi:10.1007/s00234-013-1294-y

Index

Printed in the United States
By Bookmasters